T0263597

Neonatal Nursing: Clinical Concepts and Practice Implications, Part 2

Editor

LESLIE ALTIMIER

CRITICAL CARE NURSING CLINICS OF NORTH AMERICA

www.ccnursing.theclinics.com

June 2024 • Volume 36 • Number 2

ELSEVIER

1600 John F. Kennedy Boulevard • Suite 1800 • Philadelphia, Pennsylvania, 19103-2899

http://www.theclinics.com

CRITICAL CARE NURSING CLINICS OF NORTH AMERICA Volume 36, Number 2
June 2024 ISSN 0899-5885, ISBN-13: 978-0-443-13123-3

Editor: Kerry Holland
Developmental Editor: Shivank Joshi

© **2024 Elsevier Inc. All rights are reserved, including those for text and data mining, AI training, and similar technologies.**

This periodical and the individual contributions contained in it are protected under copyright by Elsevier, and the following terms and conditions apply to their use:

Photocopying
Single photocopies of single articles may be made for personal use as allowed by national copyright laws. Permission of the Publisher and payment of a fee is required for all other photocopying, including multiple or systematic copying, copying for advertising or promotional purposes, resale, and all forms of document delivery. Special rates are available for educational institutions that wish to make photocopies for non-profit educational classroom use. For information on how to seek permission visit www.elsevier.com/permissions or call: (+44) 1865 843830 (UK)/(+1) 215 239 3804 (USA).

Derivative Works
Subscribers may reproduce tables of contents or prepare lists of articles including abstracts for internal circulation within their institutions. Permission of the Publisher is required for resale or distribution outside the institution. Permission of the Publisher is required for all other derivative works, including compilations and translations (please consult www.elsevier.com/permissions).

Electronic Storage or Usage
Permission of the Publisher is required to store or use electronically any material contained in this periodical, including any article or part of an article (please consult www.elsevier.com/permissions). Except as outlined above, no part of this publication may be reproduced, stored in a retrieval system or transmitted in any form or by any means, electronic, mechanical, photocopying, recording or otherwise, without prior written permission of the Publisher.

Notice
No responsibility is assumed by the Publisher for any injury and/or damage to persons or property as a matter of products liability, negligence or otherwise, or from any use or operation of any methods, products, instructions or ideas contained in the material herein. Because of rapid advances in the medical sciences, in particular, independent verification of diagnoses and drug dosages should be made.

Although all advertising material is expected to conform to ethical (medical) standards, inclusion in this publication does not constitute a guarantee or endorsement of the quality or value of such product or of the claims made of it by its manufacturer.

Critical Care Nursing Clinics of North America (ISSN 0899-5885) is published quarterly by Elsevier Inc., 360 Park Avenue South, New York, NY 10010-1710. Months of issue are March, June, September, and December. Business and Editorial Offices: 1600 John F. Kennedy Blvd., Suite 1800, Philadelphia, PA 19103-2899. Periodicals postage paid at New York, NY and additional mailing offices. Subscription prices are $166.00 per year for US individuals, $100.00 per year for US students and residents, $206.00 per year for Canadian individuals, $230.00 per year for international individuals, $115.00 per year for international students/residents and $100.00 per year for Canadian students/residents. For institutional access pricing please contact Customer Service via the contact information below. To receive student/resident rate, orders must be accompanied by name of affiliated institution, data of term, and the *signature* of program/residency co-ordinator on institution letterhead. Orders will be billed at individual rate until proof of status is received. Foreign air speed delivery is included in all *Clinics* subscription prices. All prices are subject to change without notice. **POSTMASTER:** Send address changes to *Critical Care Nursing Clinics of North America*, Elsevier Health Sciences Division, Subscription Customer Service, 3251 Riverport Lane, Maryland Heights, MO 63043. **Customer Service: 1-800-654-2452 (US and Canada); 314-447-8871 (outside US and Canada). Fax: 314-447-8029. E-mail:** JournalsCustomerService-usa@ elsevier.com **(for print support) and** JournalsOnlineSupport-usa@elsevier.com **(for online support).**

Reprints. For copies of 100 or more of articles in this publication, please contact the Commercial Reprints Department, Elsevier Inc., 360 Park Avenue South, New York, New York, 10010-1710; Tel.: 212-633-3874, Fax: 212-633-3820, and E-mail: reprints@elsevier.com.

Critical Care Nursing Clinics of North America is covered in *MEDLINE/PubMed (Index Medicus), International Nursing Index, Nursing Citation Index, Cumulative Index to Nursing and Allied Health Literature, and RNdex Top 100.*

Contributors

EDITOR

LESLIE ALTIMIER, DNP, RN, NE-BC, MSN, BSN
Regional Director of Neonatal Services, Cardinal Glennon Children's Hospital, St Louis, Missouri, USA

AUTHORS

LESLIE ALTIMIER, DNP, RN, NE-BC, MSN, BSN
Regional Director of Neonatal Services, Cardinal Glennon Children's Hospital, St Louis, Missouri, USA

WILLIAM CODY BARTRUG, MA, BSN, RN, RNC-NIC
Clinical Nurse II, Intensive Care Nursery, UCSF Benioff Children's Hospital, University of California, San Francisco, San Francisco, California, USA

ALLISON BEST, DNP, FNP, RN, BSN
Loma Linda University Children's Hospital, Loma Linda, California, USA

MARSHA CAMPBELL-YEO, PhD, MN, NNP-BC, RN
Full Professor and Clinician Scientist, Faculty of Health, Departments of Pediatrics and Psychology and Neuroscience, School of Nursing, Dalhousie University, MOM-LINC Lab, IWK Health, Halifax, Nova Scotia, Canada

ASHLEA D. CARDIN, OTD, OTR/L, BCP, CNT
Associate Professor of Occupational Therapy, Missouri State University, Springfield, Missouri, USA

JENNY CHU, MA, OTR/L, SWC, IBCLC
Occupational Therapist, Loma Linda University Children's Hospital, Loma Linda, California, USA

LACIE DIXON, RDCS, MHPS
Family Support Specialist, Hand to Hold, Austin, Texas, USA

ELBA FAYARD, MD
Professor, Department of Pediatrics, Division of Neonatology, Loma Linda University Medical School, Loma Linda University Children's Hospital, Loma Linda, California, USA

PAMELA A. HARRIS-HAMAN, DNP, APRN, NNP-BC
Assistant Professor, School of Nursing, University of Texas Medical Branch, Galveston, Texas, USA

CAROL B. JAEGER, DNP, RN, NNP-BC
Adjunct Faculty, The Ohio State University, Columbus, Ohio, USA

MORGAN MacNEIL, BScN, RN
PhD in Nursing Student, Faculty of Health, School of Nursing, Dalhousie University, MOM-LINC Lab, IWK Health, Halifax, Nova Scotia, Canada

YUI MATSUDA, PhD, PHNA-BC, MPH
Assistant Professor of Clinical, University of Miami School of Nursing and Health Studies, Coral Gables, Florida, USA

HELEN McCORD, BScN, RN, MN, NNP
PhD in Nursing Student, Faculty of Health, School of Nursing, Dalhousie University, MOM-LINC Lab, IWK Health, Halifax, Nova Scotia, Canada

JOY ORTIZ, BSN, RN
Registered Nurse (RN), Neonatal Intensive Care Unit, Nicklaus Children's Hospital, Miami, Florida, USA

TONYA OSWALT, RN, BSN, IBCLC
Loma Linda University Children's Hospital, Loma Linda, California, USA

CHRISTINE PEREZ, PhD, BSN, RN, CEIM
NICU Thought Leader Philips, Board of Directors, Infant Massage USA, San Diego, California, USA

RAYLENE PHILLIPS, MD, MA, IBCLC, FAAP, FABM
Associate Professor, Division of Neonatology, Department of Pediatrics, Loma Linda University Children's Hospital, Loma Linda University School of Medicine, Loma Linda, California, USA

NICOLE POLARA, MMT, MT-BC
Music Therapist II, Department of Child Life and Integrative Care, Cincinnati Children's Hospital Medical Center, Cincinnati, Ohio, USA

JAZMIN D. RAMIREZ, BSN, RN
Pre-doctoral Student, Registered Nurse (RN), University of Miami School of Nursing and Health Studies, Coral Gables, Florida, USA

PAMELA RUIZ, RN, BS, IBCLC
Loma Linda University Children's Hospital, Loma Linda, California, USA

DANIELLE ALTARES SARIK, PhD, APRN, CPNP-PC
Director of Nursing Research and Evidence-Based Practice, Nicklaus Children's Hospital, Miami, Florida, USA

JAYNE SOLOMON, MSN, APRN, NNP-BC, C-ELBW
NICU Quality Coordinator, Advanced Practice Clinical Leader, St. Joseph's Women's Hospital Neonatal Intensive Care Unit, Tampa, Florida, USA

DAWN VANNATTA, OTR/L, SWC, CNT, NTMTC, CLEC
NICU Occupational Therapist, Loma Linda University Children's Hospital, Loma Linda, California, USA

DIANNE WOOLDRIDGE, RN, IBCLC
Loma Linda University Children's Hospital, Loma Linda, California, USA

Contents

> All newborns experience pain during routine care, which can have long-lasting negative effects. Despite the availability of effective methods to prevent and reduce pain, most infants will receive ineffective or no treatment. Optimal pain management includes the reduction of the number of procedures performed, routine pain assessment and the use of effective pain-reducing interventions, most notably breastfeeding, skin-to-skin contact and sweet-tasting solutions. Parents are an essential component of the comprehensive assessment and management of infant pain; however, a gap exists regarding the uptake of parent-led interventions and the engagement of families. Practice recommendations for infant pain care are discussed.

> Substance abuse is a widespread problem in the United States and worldwide. This use within the pregnant population is thought to reflect a pattern similar to the general population, with estimates of 10% to 15% of pregnant women experiencing substance abuse. Illicit substance use during pregnancy has increased substantially during the past decade in the United States. During the past decade, novel or atypical substances have emerged and become increasingly popular. Occurrences of toxicity and untoward fetal effects from designer drug use must be kept high on the watch list for all who practice in maternal-fetal, newborn, and emergency departments.

> The increase in substance use during pregnancy results in a higher incidence of neonatal abstinence syndrome/neonatal opioid withdrawal syndrome (NAS/NOWS), straining health care and social systems and creating an economic burden. There is a paradigm shift in transitioning the care approach for NAS/NOWS from a medical model of care to a family-centered individualized non-pharmacological care approach with non-pharmacological interventions as the first line of treatment. Supporting families after birth with a nurturing environment and providing them with a toolbox of non-pharmacological interventions prepares them for the transition from hospital to home.

> The number of infants diagnosed with neonatal abstinence syndrome (NAS) or neonatal opioid withdrawal syndrome (NOWS) has increased. The expression of NAS/NOWS symptoms differs and typically begins within the first few days of life, considered a critical period for feeding skill

establishment, nourishment, and attachment. Non-pharmacologic interventions may be deployed to reduce or eliminate the need for replacement opioids while targeting outcomes like feeding dysfunction. Critical care providers can benefit from a structured examination of disordered feeding experiences to inform their selection of non-pharmacologic interventions. This structure can be provided using the Ecology of Human Performance model.

> Preterm babies who received 72 hours of breastfeeding practice before introducing a bottle had significantly higher rates of breastfeeding at the time of neonatal intensive care unit (NICU) discharge than did babies who were introduced to bottle-feeding with or before breastfeeding during the first 72 hours of oral feeding or babies who were primarily bottle-fed. There were no statistical differences in corrected gestational age (CGA) at birth, first oral feeding, or full oral feeds, in days from first to full oral feeds, or in CGA or days of life at NICU discharge.

> Mothers with an infant hospitalized in the neonatal intensive care unit (NICU) are at an increased risk of mental health concerns, including depression and anxiety. Successful mental health support during the critical time of transition from hospital to home requires careful consideration of the mothers' mental health beginning during the NICU stay. Major themes from a scoping review to identify best practices to support maternal mental health include (1) comprehensive evaluation of needs and continuity of care, (2) key role of in-person support, and (3) the potential to use technology-based support to increase mental health support.

> The death of a child is a devastating event that can lead to chronic sorrow and great stress among parents and caregivers. Legacy-building and memory-making experiences for anticipatory grief and bereavement have become increasingly popular in pediatric hospitals, including the use of heartbeat recordings. This intervention created by Brian Schreck at Cincinnati Children's Hospital Medical Center involves audio recording the patient's heartbeat or other respiratory sounds with a digital stethoscope to construct and preserve the patient's legacy, as well as to act as a therapeutic tool.

William Cody Bartrug

Parents who are experiencing neonatal death need support in promoting
and maintaining their parental role. This includes parenting their infant during end-of-life. Bedside nurses should partner with parents to help them
maintain the parent-infant relationship by establishing effective communication, building trust, and promoting the parental role. By doing so, parents will utilize these experiences to process their grief through
meaning-making.

CRITICAL CARE NURSING
CLINICS OF NORTH AMERICA

SERIES OF RELATED INTEREST

Nursing Clinics of North America http://www.nursing.theclinics.com

THE CLINICS ARE AVAILABLE ONLINE!
Access your subscription at:
www.theclinics.com

Preface

Neonatal Nursing: Clinical Concepts and Practice Implications: Part 2

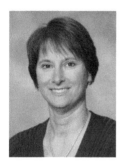

Leslie Altimier, DNP, RN, NE-BC, MSN, BSN
Editor

This issue, Part 2 of a two-part series, is once again dedicated to neonates and their families. We start this issue in the "womb" with an article by Dr Raylene Phillips titled "Bonding and Attachment with Baby in the Womb or the Neonatal Intensive Care Unit: The Critical Role of Early Emotional Connections." Both bonding and attachment can begin before birth, which impact fetal and infant brain development and may improve birth outcomes. Babies in the womb and preterm babies in the Neonatal Intensive Care Unit (NICU) can hear and respond to maternal voices with positive effects on physiologic stability and language development. Supporting emotional connections before and after birth is the responsibility and the privilege of health care providers who care for pregnant mothers and babies in the NICU.

Dr Phillips continues with a second article with authors Jayne Solomon, Lacie Dixon, and Leslie Altimier discussing "Neuroprotective Infant and Family-Centered Developmental Care for the Tiniest Babies: Perspectives from Key Members of the Neonatal Intensive Care Unit Small Baby Team." Caring for extremely preterm infants in the NICU is a multidisciplinary team effort. A clear understanding of roles for each delivery team member, anticipation of challenges, and standardized checklists support improved outcomes for this population. Physicians and nursing leaders are responsible for being role models and holding staff accountable for creating a unit culture of Neuroprotective Infant and Family-Centered Developmental Care. It is essential for parents to be included as part of the care team and for babies to be acknowledged for their efforts in coping with the developmentally unexpected NICU environment.

Crit Care Nurs Clin N Am 36 (2024) xi–xiv
https://doi.org/10.1016/j.cnc.2023.12.004
0899-5885/24/© 2023 Published by Elsevier Inc.

ccnursing.theclinics.com

The goal of baby and family-centered care is to recognize the needs of the baby exhibited through the baby's individual behavior and communication and support parent education, engagement, and interaction with the baby to build a nurturing relationship. It is essential that health care providers and caregivers guide, rather than control, the role of the parents from birth through NICU care, transition to home, and continuing care at home. Parents are members of the health care team, primary caregivers, and shared decision makers for the care of their baby. Welcome Dr Carol Jaeger as she discusses "Baby and Family-Centered Care in the Neonatal Intensive Care Unit—A Changing Perspective."

All newborns experience pain during routine care, which can have long-lasting negative effects. Despite the availability of effective methods to prevent and reduce pain, most infants will receive ineffective or no treatment. Parents are an essential component of the comprehensive assessment and management of infant pain; however, a substantial knowledge gap exists among parents surrounding effective parent-led infant pain management. Routine pain assessment is integral to evaluating the need for, as well as the efficacy of, pain-relieving interventions across different situations. In nonverbal populations, such as infants, health care providers must rely on alternative assessment methods to assist in painting a comprehensive picture of the pain experienced and subsequently achieve optimal pain management. Effective pain management is a standard of care for all infants in the NICU. The most effective method to eliminate infant pain is to reduce the number of procedures performed. Dr Marsha Campbell-Yeo, Morgan MacNeil, and Helen McCord from Halifax, Nova Scotia, Canada, share their expertise on Pain in Neonates: Perceptions and Current Practices.

Dr Pamela Harris-Haman, from the University of Texas Medical Branch, brings us an update on new opioids, psychoactive drugs, and synthetic marijuana. Substance abuse is a widespread problem in the United States and worldwide. The use within the pregnant population is believed to reflect a pattern similar to the general population, with estimates of 10% to 15% of pregnant women experiencing substance abuse. Illicit substance use during pregnancy has increased substantially over the past decade in the United States. Over the past decade, novel or atypical substances have emerged and have become increasingly popular. Recognition and treatment of new substances of abuse present many challenges for health care providers due to a lack of quantitative reporting and surveillance. Given the unknown and potentially untoward effects these substances may have on the mother and infant, health care providers need to be familiar with the potential effects of these substances on the mother, fetus, and infant when born.

We continue discussing substance abuse in pregnancy with Dr Christine Perez. The increase in substance use during pregnancy results in a higher incidence of Neonatal Abstinence Syndrome (NAS) and Neonatal Opioid Withdrawal Syndrome (NOWS) in neonates, straining health care and social systems and creating an economic burden. There is a paradigm shift in transitioning the care approach for NAS/NOWS from a medical model of care to a family-centered individualized nonpharmacologic care approach with nonpharmacologic interventions as the first line of treatment. Supporting families after birth with a nurturing environment and providing them with a toolbox of nonpharmacologic interventions prepare them for the transition from hospital to home.

Dr Ashlea Cardin from Missouri State University continues the discussion of NAS and NOWS and the impact it has on feeding. The expression of NAS/NOWS symptoms differs and typically begins within the first few days of life, considered a critical period for feeding skill establishment, nourishment, and attachment. Nonpharmacologic interventions may be deployed to reduce or eliminate the need for replacement opioids while targeting outcomes like feeding dysfunction. Critical care providers can benefit from a structured examination of disordered feeding experiences to inform their selection of nonpharmacologic interventions.

Many babies go home from the NICU without ever having breastfed directly at the mother's breast. Dr Raylene Phillips, from Loma Linda University Children's Hospital, and her team (VanNatta, Chu, Best, Ruiz, Oswalt, Wooldridge, and Fayard) describe a Quality Improvement initiative created by a multidisciplinary team (NICU physicians, lactation consultants, occupational therapists, and nurses) with the primary aim to increase the rate of preterm infants who were breastfeeding at the time of NICU discharge. A secondary aim was to determine if focusing on breastfeeding before bottle feeding would influence the time to full oral feedings or the length of hospital stay.

NICU admission and an infant's critical health condition have been strongly linked to maternal psychological distress. Parents of infants born prematurely are two times more likely to experience depressive symptoms and other mental health challenges. High levels of stress in mothers of premature infants have been correlated to elevated depressive, anxiety, and posttraumatic stress symptoms and negative maternal-infant attachment outcomes. Subsequently, the impact of poor maternal mental health on maternal-infant attachment and parenting may have longstanding negative effects. Successful mental health support during the critical time of transition from hospital to home requires careful consideration of the mothers' mental health beginning during the NICU stay. Dr Altares Sarik, Ramirez, Matsuda, and Ortiz share their scoping evaluation that reviews best practices to support maternal mental health after discharge from the NICU setting in the acute period of transition from the hospital to home.

The death of a child is a devastating event that can lead to chronic sorrow and great stress among parents and caregivers. Legacy-building and memory-making experiences for anticipatory grief and bereavement have become increasingly popular in pediatric hospitals, including the use of heartbeat recordings. Heartbeat recordings involve audio recording the patient's heartbeat or other respiratory sounds with a digital stethoscope to construct and preserve the patient's legacy, which acts as a therapeutic tool. In collaboration with the patient and/or family, recorded or live music can be combined with the heartbeat while preserving the integrity of the patient's heartbeat recording to create an opportunity for memory-making or legacy-building. From Cincinnati Children's Hospital, Nicole Polara further elaborates on this fascinating concept in her article titled "Legacy Building: The Experience of Heartbeat Recordings for Bereaved Caregivers in Pediatrics."

Parents who are experiencing neonatal death need support in promoting and maintaining their parental role. This includes parenting their infant during end-of-life. The final article of this two-part issue is written by William (Cody) Bartug from Benioff Children's Hospital in San Francisco. He reviews how attachment theory can be used as a framework to understand the dynamics of the parent-infant relationship and help foster a strong and supportive bond. Attachment theory during end-of-life care involves the recognition of the parent-infant relationship and the importance of maintaining and nurturing this bond, even in the face of a loss. By doing so, parents will utilize these experiences to process their grief through meaning-making.

It has been a privilege and an honor to be the Editor of this two-part series of scholarly articles dedicated to neonates and their families. I hope you enjoy reading the diverse topics presented.

Leslie Altimier, DNP, RN, NE-BC, MSN, BSN
Cardinal Glennon Children's Hospital
1465 South Grand Avenue
St. Louis, MO 63104, USA

E-mail address:
laltimier@gmail.com

Bonding and Attachment with Baby in the Womb or in the Neonatal Intensive Care Unit

The Critical Role of Early Emotional Connections

Raylene Phillips, MD, MA, IBCLC

KEYWORDS

- Bonding • Attachment • Fetus • Preterm • Premature infant
- Emotional connections

KEY POINTS

- Bonding and attachment are critically important for the well-being of infants and children and positively impact fetal and infant brain development.
- Bonding and attachment can begin before birth and may improve birth outcomes.
- Babies in the womb and babies born prematurely can hear and respond to maternal voices with positive effects on physiologic stability and language development.
- Supporting emotional connections before and after birth is the responsibility and the privilege of health-care providers who care for pregnant mothers and neonatal intensive care unit babies.

INTRODUCTION

The terms "bonding" and "attachment" are often used interchangeably but, technically, in psychology, bonding refers to the emotional connection of a parent-directed toward their baby or child. Attachment refers to the emotional connection of a baby or child-directed toward its primary caregiver—ideally a parent.[1]

It is important that anyone caring for infants and children understand why parent–infant bonding and attachment are so critical to the health and well-being of those in their care. Those who understand the importance of bonding and attachment will want to understand how best to support their development. Yet, these concepts are not traditionally taught in medical or nursing education or in the curriculum of most who are being trained to work with babies or children.

In the hospital, physical survival and recovery are prioritized, which of course they must be but often at the expense of mental and emotional health and well-being—the very characteristics that make us human and that largely determine the quality

Division of Neonatology, Department of Pediatrics, Loma Linda University Children's Hospital, Loma Linda University School of Medicine, 11175 Campus Street, CP 11121, Loma Linda, CA 92350, USA
E-mail address: rphillps@llu.edu

Crit Care Nurs Clin N Am 36 (2024) 157–165
https://doi.org/10.1016/j.cnc.2023.11.002
0899-5885/24/© 2023 Elsevier Inc. All rights reserved.

of our lives. Anything related to mental health is often considered to be "soft science" or even optional. We now understand, however, that we cannot separate the well-being of the mind and body, and that they are intricately connected—not just for adults but for children, newborns, and even babies in the womb.

BONDING WITH BABY IN THE WOMB

Ever since the importance of bonding and attachment has become understood, the focus has been on what happens after birth. But what if bonding and attachment can begin before birth? Is the baby in the womb capable of recognizing its mother's voice? Is the baby in the womb capable of interacting with its mother? Does it matter?

Because bonding is mother-directed, it is presumed to begin before attachment, but evidence is increasing that both can begin well before birth, at least in the third trimester. A pregnant mother can begin the bonding process of focusing on her unborn baby as soon as she learns she is pregnant. Fathers/partners, siblings, and other close family members can also begin bonding with the baby while still in the womb. It has been assumed that attachment of the baby to the mother or father can only begin after birth when we can observe the baby responding to its parents. However, there is evidence that babies in the womb can respond to their mothers, and even to their fathers if they are actively engaged in connecting to the baby before birth. In the Neonatal Intensive Care Unit (NICU), we readily see that preterm infants can respond to their parents, so it should not be a surprise to realize the same is true for the unborn baby at the same stage of "fetal" development.

Pregnant mothers often feel their unborn babies respond to talking, singing, and stroking their belly. Some wonder if their baby's response is random, whereas others are certain there is often a direct response from the baby to what their mother is doing or saying. Is the fetus capable of responding to its mother's voice heard while in the womb? Several innovative fetal studies provide evidence that it is.

Unborn babies around 33 to 34 weeks of gestation have been found to distinguish their mother's voice from an unfamiliar female voice and pure sounds, and these distinctions can be seen on functional MRI (fMRI) as differences in brain activity in auditory centers located in the temporal lobe.[2] Unborn babies whose mothers have recited a child's rhyme daily in the last few weeks of pregnancy begin to have changes in fetal heart rate when they hear their mother recite the now-familiar rhyme.[3] Fetuses have been seen on ultrasound to respond behaviorally to their mother's touch by displaying more arm, head, and mouth movements when the mothers touch their abdomen, and showing decreased arm and head movements to maternal voice.[4]

Can an unborn baby discern if its mother is speaking directly to it? A study shared at the World Association of Infant Mental Health Congress in 2006, showed that fetal heart rate variability increased (indicating a reduction of stress) significantly more when its mother communicated directly with the baby either vocally or silently, compared to when the mother talked about the fetus to another adult.[5] The ability to distinguish between their mother's communication directly to them compared to communication with someone else, is an intriguing finding. Discovering similar responses to either spoken or silent communications expands the possibilities of mother–fetus communication.

As we have seen, it is well documented that, at least in the third trimester, unborn babies can learn and remember. They learn to recognize (and prefer) their mother's voice and the words she has repeated. They also learn to recognize their father's voice or the voice of any significant other who speaks to them while they are inside the womb, and they respond to that voice after birth.[6] During this usually safe and protected time, their world is the womb and the mother who surrounds it.

What is the effect on birth outcomes when pregnant mothers focus on bonding prenatally with their unborn baby? Dr Gerhart Schroth, MD, a psychiatrist from Germany, teaches, and uses in his therapeutic practice, a program for pregnant mothers called "Prenatal Bonding, Bonding Analysis (BA), which is based on the work of Hungarian psychologist, Dr Raffai, PhD. This program supports an intense bonding between mother and baby in one-on-one weekly sessions beginning around 16 to 20 weeks of gestation. The Prenatal Bonding (BA) program helps to bring awareness and healing to any past trauma experienced by the pregnant mother, supports the mother in any current stressors, and helps the mother consciously connect with her baby in the womb. Birth becomes a partnership between mother and baby, and the mother feels she already knows her baby immediately after birth.[7]

Birth outcomes from 295 European mothers who had experienced Prenatal Bonding (BA) sessions between 2017 and 2020, when compared with the general population, showed fewer Cesarean births (18% vs 32%), fewer preterm births (2% vs 10%), increased breastfeeding rates after birth (99% vs 75%) and after 6 months (94% vs 66%), decreased rates of infantile colic (0.3% vs 20%), decreased rates of baby blues (6% vs 80%), and decreased rates of postpartum depression (0.1% vs 19%).[8]

Results from more than 8000 pregnancies using Prenatal Bonding (BA) show that preterm birth rates are consistently less than 2% (vs 9.2% in German populations). Excessive infant crying (or infantile colic) is unknown after Prenatal Bonding (BA), and postpartum depression is seen in less than 1% of mothers (vs 13%–19% in the general population) (Gerhard Schroth, MD, personal communication, 2023).

Of course, prenatal bonding is nothing new. Mothers have been talking and singing to their babies and stroking their babies inside the womb for millennia. According to the Developmental Origins of Health and Disease, "The womb may be more important than the home."[9] Prenatal bonding, in whatever way it is done, is a way to optimize the womb experience for unborn babies as well as the pregnancy experience for the mother.

BONDING WITH BABY IN THE NEONATAL INTENSIVE CARE UNIT

It is easy to forget that the preterm baby is developmentally a fetus. When we take the time to absorb this reality, it fundamentally shifts our perspective and changes our interactions with this usually perfect, but incompletely developed, tiny being in our care. The fetus and preterm infant are not ready for life outside the womb. Within the protective environment of the womb, unborn babies are free to use their developing senses to move, touch, feel, smell, taste, see, learn, and remember. Moreover, they cannot help but be connected to their mother who is their world.

The neonatal intensive care unit (NICU), of course, is nothing like the womb with no consistency in sounds, touch, or containment, and for long periods, there may be no connection with their mother—unless she is in the NICU. If the mother is physically present and emotionally available, the baby's "world" can still be the mother, and the NICU that surrounds them both will have less of a negative effect on the baby.

In Neuroprotective Infant and Family Centered Developmental Care, we make great efforts to provide a "healing environment" for the preterm or sick infant but what we must remember is that the baby's mother is the optimal healing environment, especially in the NICU. Before birth, the mother and her womb support optimal fetal development. After birth, the NICU without the mother induces stress and interrupts fetal/preterm development, but the NICU with the mother and skin-to-skin contact reduces stress and supports development, including the emotional connections of bonding and attachment.

Because prematurely born babies are in the same developmental stages as a fetus would be at the same gestational age, when exploring the possibilities in prenatal bonding, it is enlightening to review what is known about the responsiveness of preterm infants to their mother's voice and touch in the NICU. The effects of maternal voice on preterm infants in the NICU have been the focus of increasing research. A systematic review of 15 live or recorded maternal voice interventions with preterm infants in the NICU done from 2000 to 2015 found that hearing their mother's voice resulted in physiologic and behavioral stabilization with fewer cardiorespiratory events.[10]

Results of hearing their mother's voice go beyond immediate stabilization for preterm infants in the NICU. Two Italian studies have found that parental reading in the NICU positively influences language development in preterm infants at 9 months[11] and 18 months corrected gestational age (CGA).[12] A study conducted at Brown University found that preterm infants who experienced increased parental talking in the NICU had higher 7-month and 18-month corrected age Bayley-III language and cognitive scores.[13]

Exposure to the mother's voice and heartbeat was found to influence auditory plasticity in the brains of preterm infants who heard their mother's sounds for 3 hours per day for the first 30 days of life in the NICU. Preterm infants exposed to maternal sounds had a significantly larger auditory cortex bilaterally compared with control newborns receiving standard care.[2]

It has been shown that the social communication abilities of 10-year-old children can be predicted by the strength of brain connectivity in neural circuits involved in perceptions of their mother's voice as seen on fMRI. Because we have seen evidence that the fetal brain can distinguish its mother's voice, we know this process begins before birth—or in the case of the prematurely born infant, this process begins in the NICU.[14]

Some of the most intriguing studies about talking to preterm babies in the NICU have been done by Dr Betty Vohr and her team at Brown University. Dr Vohr found that as early as 32 weeks CGA, preterm infants produced vocalizations that were distinct from crying. It was also noted that preterm infants as early as 32 weeks had "conversational turns" with their parents. A conversational turn was defined as sounds by the parent or the infant within 5 seconds of each other. Both vocalizations and conversational turns were significantly increased when parents were present at their baby's bedside than when parents were absent.[15]

In the NICU, being in skin-to-skin contact is the closest preterm babies can get to being back inside the womb where they were meant to be for several more days, weeks, or months before birth. One of the many well-documented benefits of skin-to-skin contact in the NICU is improved mother–infant bonding. Mother–infant separation is a predictor of decreased bonding and attachment,[16] whereas immediate skin-to-skin contact after a preterm birth has been shown to improve bonding and attachment.[17]

If maternal presence and voice have a positive effect on premature babies in the NICU and have a positive effect on mother–infant bonding, this should also be true for unborn babies of the same gestational age of development who are fortunate enough to still be inside their mother's womb. Communication between mother and baby—born or unborn—whether verbally or silently, contributes to emotional connections, which are the basis for bonding and attachment.

We now have an increased awareness of the unborn or prematurely born baby's capacity to notice and respond to their mother's voice, and study results show the benefits for both babies and mothers in creating emotional connections as early as possible in the womb before birth—or in the NICU after a preterm birth.

IMPACT OF BONDING AND ATTACHMENT ON FETAL AND INFANT BRAIN DEVELOPMENT

Attachment has been said to have 2 basic functions: (1) ensuring that the child remains in the proximity of the primary caregiver and (2) programming the lifelong structure and function of the brain.[18] Knowledge about the critical role of experience in shaping the structure and function (even before birth) of the developing human brain has been increasing during the last several decades.[19]

Infant brain research has shown that much of brain growth, especially brain cell organization, and synaptic development, is a very active process that depends on individual experiences beginning in the womb or in the NICU, wherever the baby happens to be in the third trimester.[20,21] Dr Als and colleagues[22] demonstrated that early experiences with preterm babies in the NICU alter their brain function and structure as seen with brain imaging at 2 weeks and 9 months CGA.

Dr Schore, a neurobiologist who studies infant brain development, maintains that early experiences can positively and negatively influence the organization of the brain and that these experiences are embedded in the attachment relationship.[23] Dr Schore has proposed that the structure and function of the brain are shaped by social experiences and emotional relationships.[24] He maintains that attachment experiences specifically impact the development of the right brain, which begins a growth spurt in the last trimester of pregnancy and continues through the first year after birth.[25]

Dr Schore says, "the essential adaptive right brain functions of interdependence, social connection, and emotion regulation emerge out of early attachment experiences."[26] He suggests that the development of the emotion-processing limbic system is shaped by the mother–infant attachment relationship,[27] which we have seen can begin before birth while the baby is still in the womb or in the NICU after a premature birth.

The amygdala is part of the limbic system that is involved with emotional earning, memory modulation, and activation of the sympathetic nervous system, our fight-or-flight mechanism. The amygdala is in the midst of development in the third trimester of gestation. It is known that the fetus has well-developed senses of touch, proprioception, and smell by the third trimester. Dr Schore notes that these senses connect directly to the right amygdala in the fetal brain via the prefrontal-orbital pathway and are essential to the development of an efficiently regulated and organized right brain—beginning before birth.[24] After birth, skin-to-skin contact sends nerve impulses to the brain via the same pathway to activate the amygdala and continued development of this important part of our brain.

EMOTIONAL CONNECTIONS AS THE FOUNDATION OF BONDING AND ATTACHMENT

Nature has given every newborn the biological instinctive need for contact with its mother. For multiple reasons, skin-to-skin contact and very close proximity to their mother is the natural habitat for all newborn mammals and the optimal place for physiologic stability and for the development of the emotional connections necessary for bonding and secure attachment to occur. Skin-to-skin contact, however, is not just another location for babies to sleep. When babies are in skin-to-skin contact with their parents, the close proximity makes it easier to support an emotional connection with their baby.

The Nurture Science Program in the Columbia University Medical Center NICU is run by Dr Martha Welch, MD, and Dr Michael Myers, PhD. In this program, it is recognized that separation causes emotional trauma, and that disconnection occurs frequently. A key component of this program is to help parents and babies to reconnect each day making emotional connections by using simple interventions. Trained Nurture Specialists support mother and baby in calming sessions using the 3 simple tools of Kangaroo Care, a scent cloth, and talking to the baby. The goal is to create both a physical and emotional connection. A key feature of this intervention is that the mother and baby are always thought of together as a pair and interventional activities deliberately create emotional connections between them.

The first randomized controlled trial used this Family Nurture Intervention for only 6 hours a week, and even with this limited time frame, results at 4 months corrected age showed significantly decreased maternal anxiety and depression. At term corrected age, dramatically increased brain activity in the prefrontal cortex was seen. At 18 months, results showed significantly increased cognition and language development and a significant decrease in autism, and at 4 to 5 years, the results showed improved autonomic regulation in both mothers and children who received the Family Nurture Intervention in the NICU.[28]

The whole point of Infant and Family Centered Care is to support and build emotional connections. What happens during skin-to-skin contact—on the most fundamental level—is connection. This is what nurturing is all about, and this is the foundation for building strong bonds and secure attachments. Human connection is a basic human need and is the birthright of every new baby.

Because parental proximity is critical to building emotional connections, we must first acknowledge that parents are essential caregivers and must have 24/7 access to their NICU baby. This should be reflected in our signage, in our policies, in our language, and in our attitudes. In all of these areas, there is much room for improvement. In our signage, rather than posting "Visiting Hours are ___ to ___," how about creating signs that say, "Parents welcome to the NICU anytime. Other family members welcome from ___ to ___. Siblings welcome with Child Life appointment," or "Siblings welcome from __ to __." In our language (both verbal and documented) rather than saying, "When did parents last visit?" or writing, "Parents last visited on ___," how about asking, "When were parents last at their baby's bedside?" or "When did the parents last interact with their baby or participate in their baby's cares?" And of course, regardless of what is posted, what is said, or what is written, our attitude and behavior are of utmost importance. When speaking about parents or to parents, our body language and tone say more than any words. It is all about how we make them feel.

Because skin-to-skin contact is a critically important component in forming a baby's first connections with its mother and father outside the womb, it should not be considered an intervention—but simply a given—the most basic and most effective form of nurturing a new human being. By denying skin-to-skin contact in the NICU or making it optional, by denying parents access to their babies or making it difficult, or by denying parents the opportunities to care for their babies in the NICU, we are denying vital connections and risking short-term and long-term harm. Supporting connections in the NICU that lead to strong bonds and secure attachment as the baby develops is as critical as supporting feeding—and we have the neuroscience that tells us it is worth the investment of our time and energy.

IT IS NEVER TOO LATE FOR BONDING AND ATTACHMENT

In every NICU admission, regardless of the reason—prematurity, sepsis, or congenital condition, in many current NICUs, there is often a break in the bonding/attachment process that results in emotional wounds for mothers and babies. Having your baby in the NICU is on no one's birth plan, and the very nature of having a baby who needs intensive care is, at the very least, unexpected and disruptive and at worst, can be terrifyingly disabling. That's the bad news.

The good news is that the wounds of disrupted bonding can be healed. If the wound is acknowledged, it can be healed, and even if bonding and attachment are completely missed in the neonatal period, they can be developed at any time in a baby, child, or even adult's life. However, it is so much easier when it begins before birth and during the newborn period when babies' brains are developmentally primed to make emotional connections that form strong bonds and secure attachments with their parents.

SUMMARY

NICU health-care providers, whose job is to provide the best possible whole-baby care for NICU babies, must understand the critical importance of bonding and attachment for optimal infant physical, cognitive, and emotional growth and development. Parent–infant bonding must be made a priority by supporting parental proximity, skin-to-skin contact, and the development of emotional connections at every opportunity.

Those who care for pregnant mothers, whose job is to provide the best possible whole-mother/fetal care should understand that bonding and attachment can begin before birth. They must be aware that prenatal bonding has the potential to improve birth outcomes for both the mother and baby. Pregnant mothers may not be aware that their unborn baby can hear and respond to their voice or thoughts, and health-care providers taking care of pregnant mothers can support them in ways to interact with their unborn baby—by talking, singing, or communicating silently to their baby, or by touching and stroking their baby through their belly and noticing any responses.

Evidence has been building for many years that bonding and attachment in the womb, in the hospital, in the birthing center, and in the home are critically important to the growth, development, health, and well-being of all babies. It is our responsibility and privilege to share this information and support this process for the babies and mothers in our care and for the families that support them.

CLINICS CARE POINTS

- Supporting bonding and attachment must be prioritized to support the well-being of infants and children and optimal fetal and infant brain development.

- Pregnant mothers can interact with their babies before birth, knowing their unborn babies in the womb can hear and respond to their voices and touch.

- Parents of NICU babies can be supported in talking with their preterm babies, knowing that hearing their parents' voices enhances physiologic stability, brain development, and language development.

- Although bonding and attachment are possible at any time during the life span, they are more easily developed in the fetal and neonatal period when the human brain is primed for the establishment of early connections.

ACKNOWLEDGMENTS

The author wishes to acknowledge, with gratitude, the work of the Association for Prenatal and Perinatal Psychology and Health (APPPAH), a global nonprofit organization that has studied Birth Psychology for more than 40 years. APPPAH's mission is to provide education about prenatal and perinatal sciences for birth professionals and parents to help prevent birth trauma and promote the development of healthy emotional connections before and after birth. More information can be found at www.birthpsychology.com.

DISCLOSURE

The author has no commercial or financial conflicts of interest, no funding sources, and no disclosures to make.

REFERENCES

1. Ettenberger M, Bieleninik Ł, Epstein S, et al. Defining attachment and bonding: overlaps, differences, and implications for music therapy clinical practice and research in the neonatal intensive care unit (NICU). Int J Environ Res Publ Health 2021;18(4):1733.
2. Webb AR, Heiler HT, Benson CB, et al. Mother's voice and heartbeat sounds elicit auditory plasticity in the human brain before full gestations. Proc Natl Acad Sci U S A 2015;112(10):3152–7.
3. DeCasper J, Lecanuet JP, Busnel MC, et al. Fetal reactions to recurrent maternal speech. Infant Behav and Dev 1994;17(2):159–64.
4. Marx V, Nagy E. Fetal behavioural responses to maternal voice and touch. PLoS One 2015;10(6):e0129118.
5. Marie-Claire B, Thierry V, Aurélie R, et al. Communication between mother and infant (fetus or newborn). World association of infant mental health - WAIMH congress, 2006, Paris, France. Infant Ment Health J 2006;27(3A):738. Supplement to the Infant Mental Health Journal. ⟨hal-01598660⟩.
6. Lee GY, Kisilevsky BS. Fetuses respond to father's voice but prefer mother's voice after birth. Dev Psychobiol 2014;56(1):1–11.
7. Schroth G. Introduction to prenatal bonding (BA). In: Evertz K, Janus L, Linder R, editors. Handbook of prenatal and perinatal psychology. Switzerland: Springer Nature; 2021. p. 595–8.
8. Goertz-Schroth A, Schroth G, Phillips R. Prenatal Bonding (BA) as a breakthrough in improving pregnancy, birth, and postpartum outcomes. JOPPPAH 2023; 37(1):6–27.
9. Nicoletto SF, Rinaldi A. In the womb's shadow. The theory of prenatal programming as the fetal origin of various adult diseases is increasingly supported by a wealth of evidence. EMBO Rep 2011;12(1):30–4.
10. Filippa M, Panza C, Ferrari F, et al. Systematic review of maternal voice interventions demonstrates increased stability in preterm infants. Acta Paediatr 2017; 106(8):1220–9.
11. Neri E, De Pascalis L, Agostini F, et al. Parental book-reading to preterm born infants in NICU: the effects on language development in the first two years. Int J Environ Res Publ Health 2021;18(21):11361.
12. Biasini A, Fantini F, Neri E, et al. Communication in the neonatal intensive care unit: a continuous challenge. J Matern Fetal Neonatal Med 2012;25:2126–9.
13. Caskey M, Stephens B, Tucker R, et al. Adult talk in the NICU with preterm infants and developmental outcomes. Pediatrics 2014;133(3):e578–84.
14. Abrams DA, Chen T, Odriozola P, et al. Neural circuits underlying mother's voice perception predict social communication abilities in children. Proc Natl Acad Sci USA 2016;113(22):6295–300.

15. Caskey M, Stephens B, Tucker R, et al. Importance of parent talk on the development of preterm infant vocalizations. Pediatrics 2011;128(5):910–6.
16. Darvishvand M, Khalesi ZB, Rahebi SM. Mother-infant relationship and its predictors. JBRA Assist Reprod 2022;26(1):68–72.
17. Lilliesköld S, Zwedberg S, Linnér A, et al. Parents' experiences of immediate skin-to-skin contact after the birth of their very preterm neonates. J Obstet Gynecol Neonatal Nurs 2022 Jan;51(1):53–64.
18. Sullivan RM. The neurobiology of attachment to nurturing and abusive caregivers. Hastings Law J 2012 Aug;63(6):1553–70.
19. Tierney AL, Nelson CA 3rd. Brain development and the role of experience in the early years. Zero Three 2009;30(2):9–13.
20. Luis Bettio L, Thacker JS, Hutton C, et al. Chapter twelve - modulation of synaptic plasticity by exercise. In: Suk-Yu Y, Kwok-Fai S, editors. International review of neurobiology147. Academic Press; 2019. p. 295–322.
21. Kolb B, Mychasiuk R, Muhammad A, et al. Experience and the developing prefrontal cortex. Proc Natl Acad Sci USA 2012;109(Suppl 2):17186–93.
22. Als Heidelise, PhD, Als H, et al. Early experience alters brain function and structure. Pediatrics 2004;113(4):846–57.
23. Schore AN. The effects of early relational trauma on right brain development, affect regulation, and infant mental health. Infant Ment Health J 2001;22(1–2):201–69.
24. Schore AN. The experience-dependent maturation of a regulatory system in the orbital prefrontal cortex and the origin of developmental psychopathology. Dev Psychopathol 1996;8:59–87.
25. Schore AN. Affect regulation and the origin of the self. The neurobiology of emotional development. Mahwah, NJ: Erlbaum; 1994.
26. Schore AN. Early interpersonal neurobiological assessment of attachment and autistic spectrum disorders. Front Psychol 2014;5:1049.
27. Schore AN. Attachment, affect regulation, and the developing right brain: linking developmental neuroscience to pediatrics. Pediatr Rev 2005;26:204–12.
28. Welch MG, Barone JL, Porges SW, et al. Family nurture intervention in the NICU increases autonomic regulation in mothers and children at 4-5 years of age: follow-up results from a randomized controlled trial. PLoS One 2020;15(8):e0236930.

Neuroprotective Infant and Family-Centered Developmental Care for the Tiniest Babies

Perspectives from Key Members of the Neonatal Intensive Care Unit Small Baby Team

Raylene Phillips, MD, MA, IBCLC[a,*],
Jayne Solomon, MSN, APRN, NNP-BC, C-ELBW[b], Lacie Dixon, RDCS, MHPS[c],
Leslie Altimier, DNP, RN, NE-BC, MSN, BSN[d]

KEYWORDS

- ELBW • NICU • Neuroprotective • Small baby • Developmental care • Physician
- Nurse • Parent

KEY POINTS

- Physicians: Daily rounds are opportunities to be role models for Neuroprotective Infant and Family-Centered Developmental Care practices in patient care and family involvement.
- Nursing and Staff: For a small baby delivery team, anticipation, standardized checklists, and role definition are key to supporting a smooth transition from intrauterine to extra-uterine life for extremely preterm babies.
- Nursing Leadership: Accountability for consistent care standards is essential for creating a unit culture of Neuroprotective Infant and Family-Centered Developmental Care.
- Parents: It is essential to be included as part of the care team.
- Babies: Every encounter with a small baby is an opportunity to acknowledge their efforts to grow and mature in the developmentally unexpected neonatal intensive care unit environment.

[a] Loma Linda University Children's Hospital, Loma Linda University School of Medicine, 11175 Campus Street, CP 11121, Loma Linda, CA 92350, USA; [b] St. Joseph's Women's Hospital Neonatal Intensive Care Unit, 10336 Carol Cove Place, Tampa, FL 33612, USA; [c] Hand to Hold, 12325 Hymeadow Suite 4-102, Austin, TX 78750, USA; [d] SCardinal Glennon Children's Hospital, 1465 South Grand Avenue, St. Louis, MO 63104, USA
* Corresponding author.
E-mail address: rphillps@llu.edu

Crit Care Nurs Clin N Am 36 (2024) 167–184
https://doi.org/10.1016/j.cnc.2023.11.003
0899-5885/24/© 2023 Elsevier Inc. All rights reserved.

INTRODUCTION

Caring for extremely low birth weight (ELBW) infants (<1000 g at birth) involves many challenges, including ethical dilemmas regarding when to offer perinatal monitoring and resuscitation, reaching consensus in the development of policies and guidelines, creating motivation from physicians and staff to follow them, and monitoring outcomes to determine their effectiveness. Medical care for ELBW infants requires advanced knowledge of the complex physiology of fragile infants who are in "fetal" stages of development and whose medical needs can change suddenly and frequently.

Providing Neuroprotective Infant and Family-Centered Developmental Care (NIFCDC) in the neonatal intensive care unit (NICU) for any baby is a multidisciplinary team effort, especially when caring for the smallest of preterm infants. Each member of the NICU team has a role, and each role comes with a unique perspective. At the 36th Annual Gravens Conference on the Environment of Care for High-Risk Neonates held in Clearwater, Florida, in March of 2023, a workshop was held on "Neuroprotective Small Baby Care" with a focus on various perspectives of the NICU team, including physicians, staff and nursing, nursing leadership, parent, and baby. This article introduces the person who represented each role and describes the perspectives shared at the Gravens workshop on NIFCDC for the tiniest NICU babies.

PHYSICIAN PERSPECTIVES

Raylene Phillips, MD, MA, IBCLC, FAAP, FABM, raised three children and cared for nearly 2 dozen foster babies before earning an MA in developmental psychology and attending medical school. She is an International Board-Certified Lactation Consultant (IBCLC) and was Newborn Individualized Developmental Care and Assessment Program (NICDCAP) Certified as a preterm infant developmental specialist before training to be a neonatologist at Loma Linda University Children's Hospital (LLUCH) in Loma Linda, California. She is currently the Pediatric Department Chair and the Medical Director of Neonatal Services at the Loma Linda University Medical Center-Murrieta in Murrieta, California. She was the codirector of the Neuro-NICU at LLUCH and was instrumental in creating a Tiny Baby Program, which opened in 2018.

Physicians create medical policies and procedures in the NICU and have a unique opportunity to help shape the NICU environment and culture to support the optimal physical and emotional health of babies, parents, and staff. The principles and practices of NIFCDC are not part of the medical school curriculum, so physicians need education about the evidence that consistent practice of NIFCDC makes a positive difference in outcomes.[1–3] Similarly, the importance of nurture in early life and the need for newborn infants to continue the early bonds of connections with their mother begun in the womb are also not a subject given priority in medical education.

Physicians need evidence-based education as much as any other NICU staff. Ideally, there will be a physician champion who understands the medical importance of NIFCDC and can share this information with their colleagues. Once they have the evidence, physicians have a responsibility to model NIFCDC practices and to demonstrate that consistency and collaboration in this model of care are paramount. Dr Phillips shares her perspective on the physician's role in promoting and supporting NIFCDC for the smallest NICU babies.

WHY IS A FOCUS ON THE SMALL BABY POPULATION NEEDED?

- ELBW infants are more vulnerable due to their extreme prematurity and are at significantly increased risk for higher rates of mortality and morbidity. It has

been demonstrated that outcomes are improved when this population is cared for with collaborative interdisciplinary standardized care models.[4]
- Nationwide Children's Hospital was the first in the United States to demonstrate that standardized care was one of the critical components to improving morbidity and mortality of ELBW infants.[5]

HOW DO SMALL BABIES' NEUROPROTECTIVE DEVELOPMENTAL CARE NEEDS DIFFER FROM LARGER BABIES?

- Because of their extreme prematurity, they need the key aspects of NIFCDC to be practiced with even more consistency than larger babies.
- It is even more important that their physical examinations and cares are:
  - Done gently with slow movements
  - Supported by another staff member in two-person cares
  - Scheduled around care/touch times to protect sleep
- It is even more important that their healing environment includes:
  - A quiet atmosphere with protection from loud voices and other noises to safeguard their newly developing hearing senses and to protect sleep
  - Individual dim lighting with protection from bright direct light to safeguard their immature eyes
  - Soft boundaries to provide comfort and support flexed containment
- It is even more important that their mother/parent be supported in being present for:
  - Early, frequent, and prolonged skin-to-skin contact
  - Developmentally appropriate interaction, including soft talking or singing
  - Establishment of emotional connections between baby and mother/parent

HOW CAN PHYSICIANS RESPECTFULLY AND SENSITIVELY COMMUNICATE WITH BABIES, PARENTS, AND STAFF?

- When talking with babies, the physician can:
  - Use a soft, soothing voice
  - Introduce themselves and tell the baby what they are about to do before touching the baby.
  - Apologize for the cold hard stethoscope before gently touching the baby's chest with it.
  - Apologize for any uncomfortable or painful procedure
  - Tell the baby when they are finished with the examination or procedure
- When talking with parents, the physician can:
  - Sit down on a chair whenever possible
  - Use parents' language of choice and get an interpreter if needed
  - Ask how they want to be addressed (first or last name, what pronouns?)
  - Use their baby's name and correct pronoun
  - Involve parents in medical rounds and discussions about care. Avoid medical jargon
  - Ask how they think their baby is doing and if they have any observations, concerns, questions, or suggestions
  - Value and respect what parents have to say about their baby or the NICU experience
  - Encourage and support the use of mother's milk if appropriate for the baby
  - Encourage and support skin-to-skin holding whenever possible
  - Encourage and support soft talking, singing, or reading to their baby

    ○ Ask for any ideas about ways to support parents better
- When talking with NICU staff, the physician can:
  - Model the healing environment they want staff to provide
  - Use a very soft voice when talking to staff at the bedside
  - Ask the baby's nurse when care/touch times are before doing examinations
  - Do examinations only with nurse or staff support in two-person cares
  - Include them in medical rounds
  - Ask for their perspective on care plans
  - Ask for any questions, concerns, or suggestions
  - Ask if there is anything the staff member needs before moving on to the next patient

STAFF AND NURSING PERSPECTIVES

Jayne Solomon, MSN, APRN, NNP-BC, C-ELBW, has been involved in the NICU for over 30 years, serving in many capacities, including bedside care, leadership, and transport. Currently, she is working as an evidence-based practice specialist in the NICU at St Joseph's Women's Hospital (SJWH) in Tampa, Florida. Jayne is the coordinator of the small baby team, expert intravenous (IV) team, and cooling program. She enjoys building teams and participating at the bedside in the implementation of new initiatives.

Nurses and therapists (respiratory, physical, and occupational therapy) are essential to the medical care of NICU patients and also to the consistent practice of NIFCDC. They are the "eyes and ears" of physicians who care for multiple patients and cannot be at the bedside of any one baby all day or night. For NIFCDC to be effective, it must be consistent. Although physicians write medical and care orders, it is nurses and therapists who implement that care, and it is how they do it that makes the difference between short- and long-term outcomes known to result from NIFCDC. NIFCDC is a philosophy of care. It is as much about pacing, intention, and the energy the care provider brings to the bedside as it is about technique. Nurses and therapists need education about NIFCDC principles and practices, and they also must have the inner motivation to provide care in a manner that is gentle and sensitive to the baby's individual and frequently fluctuating behavioral and physiologic cues.

To be most effective, NIFCDC must begin at the moment of birth, not after the baby has been stabilized. The delivery process is improved with clearly defined roles, anticipation of known challenges, and checklists to ensure uniformity of care, avoid confusion, and reduce redundancy or omission of critical care practices. Jayne Solomon, an experienced bedside nurse and neonatal nurse practitioner (NNP), shares what the NICU small baby team at her hospital has learned in their efforts to improve the transition from intrauterine to extrauterine life for ELBW babies in the delivery room.

ST JOSEPH'S WOMEN'S HOSPITAL NEONATAL INTENSIVE CARE UNIT

- Level IV NICU, located in Tampa, FL
- Approximately 6000 deliveries/year
- 200 team members
- 24-hour house coverage: neonatologists, NNPs, physician assistants (PAs)
- 24-hour in-house pediatric transport team
- Dedicated therapeutic hypothermia team
- Dedicated expert vascular access team

- Dedicated small baby team for ELBW infants $\leq$ 27 6/7 weeks, $\leq$ 1000 g

DEVELOPING A SMALL BABY TEAM REQUIRES

- Emphasis on intentional and expeditious care of the newly born small baby
- Recognition that every tiny thing matters to the small baby

SMALL BABY PROGRAM COMPONENTS

- Pre-flight roles and responsibilities checklist
- Golden hour reminder checklist in special delivery unit
- Prenatal review checklist
- Admission checklist
- Small baby bedside binder
- 1:1 small baby team nurse for the first 72 hours of life
- Small baby team nurse for the first 21 days of life

MULTIDISCIPLINARY COLLABORATION FOR THE MANAGEMENT OF THE EXTREMELY LOW BIRTH WEIGHT INFANT

- Efforts to improve patient outcomes are often centered on mock scenarios with clearly defined participant roles.
- The cornerstone of the Neonatal Resuscitation Program (NRP) refers to each team member understanding their role and clear communication among team members.
- This same principle of team member synchrony during delivery and resuscitation can be applied to the care of the ELBW infant in the NICU.
- ELBW infants require a multidisciplinary approach that is standardized and well-coordinated among providers and team members.

ANTICIPATING A HIGH-RISK DELIVERY

- Anticipation of delivery is the first step in the management of the ELBW infant.
- Collaboration with obstetrics (OB) and labor and delivery (L&D) is important to ensure a smooth transition from intrauterine to extrauterine life.
- This can be accomplished using situation, background, assessment, recommendation (SBAR) reporting among the OB/L&D Charge Registered Nurse (RN), NICU Charge RN, transport team lead, and administrator on duty for the shift.

SMALL BABY ALERT IS TREATED AS LIKE A TRAUMA ALERT

- A small baby alert is sent before each small baby delivery and alerts the team to immediately begin preparations for delivery attendance and admission.
  - "Small Baby Alert! Only emergent calls to Neo/Neonatal nurse practitioner (NNP)/Charge RN for the next 90 minutes, please."
- When the ELBW admission is viewed as a trauma alert or rapid response (for unanticipated deliveries), a standardized approach to care that includes all NICU disciplines and support personnel is viewed as the highest priority. *This is the first critical step to improving outcomes for this population.*
- The small baby alert is sent to all NICU team members who will be both directly and indirectly involved in the admission of the infant. This includes pharmacy, radiology, respiratory, and other team members in the immediate area of the assigned bed for admission.

- The small baby alert allows the admitting nurse time to hand off her current patients and respiratory therapist (RT) to prepare the room with anticipated equipment.

PREFLIGHT CHECKLIST

- Before the admission of a small baby, a preflight checklist will be reviewed. This checklist highlighting each role and its responsibilities can easily be shared by all disciplines to ensure clear communication and collaboration.
- The charge nurse distributes the preflight checklist (six copies: one for each role)
  ○ Charge RN, admitting RN, charge RT, admitting RT, Neo/NNP, hospital unit clerk

ON ARRIVAL TO THE DELIVERY ROOM

- The golden hour reminder checklist is located in the special delivery unit.
- The team should have a brief huddle regarding the management of the anticipated infant.
- Roles are reviewed and the delivery bed is set up according to NRP standards.
- Time permitting, the charge nurse will huddle with the delivery neonatologist to make admission plans that are individualized to the anticipated needs of the infant. This might include the mode of administration of surfactant: using the endotracheal tube or by the less invasive surfactant administration.

DELIVERY ROOM HUDDLE IN THE DELIVERY ROOM

- Dedicated delivery team: Provider (Neo/NNP/PA), RT, RN
- Warmer baby alert for babies ≤ 32 weeks gestational age (GA)
- Midline head positioner

DELIVERY ROOM ACTIVITIES

- Golden hour goal: The delivery nurse obtains head circumference, length, and weight, and places oral gastric tube, whereas RT sets up equipment.
- The head of the bed (HOB) is elevated during resuscitation and transport.
- L&D or operating room (OR) staff to obtain placental laboratories. This includes a cord gas, type and screen, and blood culture for all small babies. Placental surface cultures are also obtained.

Before Leaving the Delivery Room

- The delivery RN will call report to the charge RN and RT in the NICU.
- This collaboration ensures the admitting room is set up with the correct ventilatory equipment, anticipated fluids, and any requested drugs.
- Because the pharmacy is included in the small baby alert, they are ready to provide additional drips and medications.
- Because radiology is included in the small baby alert, they will be available at the bedside for endotracheal tube confirmation and line placement.

Critical Roles at the Time of Admission

- Neonatologist, NNP/PA, delivery RN, delivery RT, admitting RN, admitting RT, scribe who also serves as the door manger (baby bouncer), and family attendant

- Two of the most important roles of the small baby admission are the family attendant and the scribe.
  - Family attendant:
    - Many times, the mother's partner will accompany the infant to the NICU.
    - This person can get lost in the admission process.
    - It is very important to have an assigned team member to update the family member and escort them back to mom or a waiting area. This is usually the nurse who attended the delivery.
  - Scribe/door manager (baby bouncer):
    - This should be a strong, experienced member of the small baby team who is familiar with the goals of the golden hour.
    - The scribe is responsible for calling the first time out when the delivery team arrives at the admitting room.
    - During the golden hour of admission, the scribe's location is the entryway of the admission room. The scribe serves as a traffic controller and as a resource for any additional items or phone calls.
- The roles of the patient care technologist, lactation consultant, and unit secretary are also critical components of the ELBW infant admission team.
  - Patient care technologist
    - Maintains a pre-stocked, prewarmed giraffe bed set on hold.
  - Lactation team
    - Notified by a "Code Gold" and prioritizes working with mom to hand express first colostrum milk drops to be used for oral care or initial tropic feeding.
  - Unit secretary
    - Promptly enters the small baby into the NICU admission base to ensure team members can input orders without delay.
- Although collaboration is key to a successful admission, it is important to only have team members in the room who have an assigned role.
  - Overcrowding leads to increased noise, too many hands on the infant, and possible contamination of any sterile equipment such as umbilical line trays.

THE SMALL BABY ADMIT CHECKLIST: COMPLETED BY THE SCRIBE

- Patient name, time of birth, time of, data from three golden hour huddles and a debriefing huddle after the golden hour
  - At SJWH, the golden hour begins when the baby arrives to the NICU room after being transported from the delivery room where a brief resuscitation has occurred.
- Admit time-out huddle—called by the scribe on admission to the NICU patient room after delivery:
  - The Neo/NNP describes the flow of the admission including:
    - The order of procedures (surfactant administration, central lines, respiratory settings, fluid rates), and anything else needed at the bedside.
    - Time outs are called at 15 and 30 minutes for temperature checks by the scribe
- At the 30-minute time out—The team discusses if the initial admitting plan needs to be adjusted and if the team is on track to get dextrose, surfactant, and antibiotics delivered by 60 to 90 minutes of life.
  - The scribe leads the discussion regarding a peripheral IV (PIV) attempt to begin glucose infusion if the provider has not established central line access.

- o The scribe is responsible for monitoring the infant's vital signs (per monitor) while entering information in the electronic medical record (EMR).
- o The scribe reminds the bedside nurse to check the infant's temperature at 15-minute intervals to ensure normothermia (a critical part of the scribe's responsibility).
  - ▪ The plastic bag, warming mattress, and servo control should all be addressed.
- o The scribe is the traffic controller of the room. The scribe ensures that all team members in the room are completing their assigned responsibilities in their roles and no additional team members are in the room who do not have a role.
- o The scribe is responsible for ensuring a smooth golden hour admission and for ensuring that the bedside incubator top down at 90 minutes.
- 60-minute time out—called by the scribe
  - o Do we need to adjust any plans?
  - o Did we get dextrose, surfactant, and antibiotic started by 60 to 90 minutes of life or at what hour of life (HOL)?
- A golden hour debrief—held after the golden hour
  - o Attended by: Admitting Neo and NNP/PA, delivery RN and RT, admitting RN and RT, charge RN and RT, small baby backup RN, and pharmacist
  - o Golden hour wins are identified as well as areas of concern and recommendations for changes
  - o Any identified process issues will be communicated to the appropriate department for review and modification if needed.

SMALL BABY GOLDEN HOUR (STARTS AT THE TIME THE BABY ARRIVES IN THE NEONATAL INTENSIVE CARE UNIT ROOM)

- Strive for golden hour management that mimics the golden hour of trauma.
- This takes time and practice!
- Always maintain excellent communication.

GOLDEN HOUR GOALS FOR FIRST 60 TO 90 MINUTES OF LIFE: LISTED ON SMALL BABY ADMISSION CHECKLIST

- Continuous temperature surveillance, prevent swings in temperature, document any drastic change in patient temperature
- Humidity set at 75% to 80%, place incubator top down by 90 minute: Time_____
- Head-to-toe skin assessment performed as a team, adequate barrier in place
- No band-aids in use, minimize adhesive
- Surfactant administered by 30 minute: Time_____
- Dextrose infusing within 60 minute ($\leq$2 PIV attempts): Time _____
- Central lines placed: Time _____, UA/UV fluids started: Time_____
- Mode of ventilation is adequate for the infant's oxygenation, gas exchange, and work of breathing
- Tortle in place, HOB elevated, eye/ear protection in use (Tortle, hat, muffs, bili mask)
- Two-person cares throughout the golden hour
- Mom updated; colostrum collection kit provided: Time_____
- Provide family the opportunity to obtain photos and touch the infant
- Fluconazole ordered if the infant is < 750 g
- Blood culture ordered: Time_____, Blood culture obtained: Time_____
- Ampicillin ordered: Time_____, Ampicillin given: Time_____

- Gentamicin ordered: Time_____, Gentamicin given: Time_____
- Admit to NICU by 30 to 90 minute: Time_____
- Huddle with the care team once the infant is stable
- Complete the golden hour wins sheet

SMALL BABY PLACENTAL LABORATORY GUIDE

- Placental blood cultures are obtained by L&D/OR team
  - Obtain cord blood, cord drug screen, cord blood gases
  - Obtain placental surface culture swab, placental blood culture, placental tissue pathology
- Each laboratory includes:
  - Drawn by _____
  - Hand-off to _____
  - Ordered by_____
  - Results in (mom's/baby's) chart

COMMUNICATION

- Ongoing communication is required between the delivery RN and the L&D RN in attendance.
- Communication should include plans for delayed cord clamping, cord blood collection, and updated information regarding the status of the mother and baby.
- Simultaneously, the NICU team should ensure all preparations are complete for the infant's admission.
- Time permitting, a small baby prenatal information sheet should be started by the NICU admitting nurse with the goal of completing the sheet before admission if possible.
  - Includes prenatal risk factors
  - Ensures that the admitting nurse is aware of significant maternal history that may inform care plans for the baby.
  - Assists in completing the EMR admission database

SMALL BABY PRENATAL INFO SHEET (A BABY'S STORY BEGINS IN UTERO)

- Infection Prevention
  - Prolonged rupture of membranes (ROM) (# of hours___, # of days___)
  - Maternal COVID-19 illness at any point during pregnancy
  - Maternal Group B *Streptococcus* (GBS) positive or unknown
  - Maternal fever during labor
  - Maternal antibiotics greater than 4 hours before delivery
  - Diagnosis of chorioamnionitis
  - Maternal infections (Hepatitis B [Hep B], Hepatitis C [Hep C], human immunodeficiency virus [HIV], Herpes, Syphilis, and Chlamydia & Gonorrhea [C/G])
  - Unexpected preterm labor or premature rupture of membranes
  - Placenta sent for culture of pathology (f/u results in 5–7 days)
- Skin/Thermoregulation
  - Placental abruption or other conditions that would expose skin to blood fluid
  - Maternal fungal infection
  - Small for gestational age (SGA)
- Nutrition

- o Intrauterine growth restriction (high-risk for neonatal feed intolerance)
- o Enhanced fetal growth - large for gestational age (LGA)
- o Maternal diabetes: Type_____
- o Cord abnormality (abnormal insertion, two-vessel, absent, or reverse flow)
- o Placental abnormality (previa, subchorionic hemorrhage, marginal insertion, velamentous cord insertion, abruption)
- Neurodevelopmental
  - o Magnesium sulfate during labor for neuroprotection
  - o In-utero exposure to drugs/alcohol
  - o Maternal hypertension
  - o Hemolysis, Elevated liver enzymes, Low platelet count (HELLP Syndrome)
  - o Preeclampsia
  - o Placental abruption, fetomaternal hemorrhages, significant anemia
  - o Significant maternal event (code, seizures, and so forth)
  - o ABO incompatibility or Rhesus (RH) incompatibility
  - o Biophysical profile score ____/____
- Respiratory
  - o Betamethasone injections (Dates:_____ _____)
  - o Oligohydramnios or anhydramnios
- Family
  - o Adequate prenatal care
  - o Maternal history of anxiety or depression
  - o Previous loss or child with diabetes
  - o History of suspected/actual abuse
  - o Requires/requests language interpreter

SMALL BABY LESSONS LEARNED

- Lesson 1: Define Roles
  - o Before admission, review roles and responsibilities.
  - o No students or interns within the patient room until after golden hour is complete.
  - o The scribe must be a strong nurse to assist with the strict golden hour timeline and to control noise and crowd traffic in and out of the delivery room (baby bouncer).
  - o The scribe should be a team member who is very comfortable with Small Baby goals.
  - o A scribe should be someone who can dedicate the first 90 minutes to being at the bedside.
- Lesson 2: Expect Revisions
  - o Initial admit RN assessment is focused on the safe transfer of the baby from the delivery room, attaching the infant to NICU monitors, and temperature control.
  - o Obtain a quick set of vitals [temperature, heart rate, respiratory rate, oxygen saturation, blood pressure (x1)].
  - o Immediately prioritize lines and surfactant (after team discussion with Neo/NNP/PA).
  - o During line/surfactant preparation, if there is an extra moment, provide newborn medications. Otherwise, defer until after line placement.
  - o Defer four-extremity blood pressures, chest/abdomen circumference
- Lesson 3: Golden Hour Time Out Huddles

○ Neonatologist (Neo) or Team Leader calls "Golden Hour Time-Out" on arrival to the delivery room: communicates plan.
○ Scribe calls "Golden Hour Time-Out" at 30 minute of life: Do we need to adjust the plan, are we on track to get dextrose, surfactant, and antibiotics in by hour of life (HOL) 1?
○ Scribe calls "Golden Hour Time-Out" at 60 minute of life: Do we need to adjust plans, did we get dextrose, surfactant, and antibiotic started by HOL 1?
○ Neo/charge RN calls for golden hour debrief after the baby is settled, the incubator top is down, and the team is available: The team fills out the reverse side of the small baby admit checklist (documents golden hour wins).
- Lesson 4: Team Member Ongoing Education
  ○ Intravenous (IV) fluids should be hung and flushed through the IV tubing before the baby gets to NICU and is ready to connect as soon as the MD/NNP is comfortable with line placement.
    ■ Do not wait for suturing.
  ○ HOB should be elevated at all times.
  ○ NeoWrap should be over the baby when drapes are removed and before putting the top down to ensure temperature stability.
  ○ Ampicillin (first antibiotic) should be started within HOL 1, after cultures are obtained.
- Lesson 5: Debrief ASAP, Individualize Baby Cares, and Celebrate the Wins
  ○ Once golden hour is complete and the infant is stable, a golden hour debrief huddle should be performed with Neo/NNP/Charge/RN/Staff RN/RT to review the reverse side of the small baby admit checklist (golden hour wins).
  ○ Prepare a small baby bedside binder for each small baby.
  ○ Prepare a small baby cart for each small baby's bedside for small baby supplies.
  ○ Celebrate the wins!
    ■ Graduation cap and gown for each small baby discharge.
    ■ Special cake or food for small baby team wins.

NURSING LEADERSHIP PERSPECTIVES

Leslie Altimier, DNP, MSN, BSN, RNC, NEA-BC, is currently the Regional Director of Neonatal Services for sisters of St. Marys (SSM) Health (Cardinal Glennon Children's Hospital and St Mary's Hospital) in St Louis, MO. She is also the Editor-in-Chief for the Journal of Neonatal Nursing, the official journal of the Neonatal Nurses Association in the United Kingdom. In her 30-plus-year nursing career, Leslie has worked clinically, in executive leadership roles, as well as in industry. Dr Altimier is a renowned clinician who lectures internationally and has published over 200 articles, chapters, and books on topics related to the clinical care of neonates, neuroprotective family-centered developmental care, NICU design, NICU of the future, and organizational leadership. Dr Altimier shares her perspective on the leader's role in creating a culture of change for health care professionals worldwide.

Nursing leadership in the NICU can make or break the culture of NIFCDC. Without nursing leadership support, education will not be prioritized, and principles and practices will not be supported. It is the responsibility of nursing leadership to provide clear job descriptions and expectations for NIFCDC when hiring new nurses, to provide initial and annual education about NIFCDC principles and practices, and the philosophy of NIFCDC, and then to hold nurses accountable for consistently putting into practice what is learned about NIFCDC care. Nursing school curriculums do not typically emphasize the critically important role of parents in the care of hospitalized infants and children. When hiring new nurses, it is important to screen for attitudes about parents and their role in the NICU and to foster a culture of including parents as active members of the care team for their NICU babies. Leslie Altimier shares what she has learned in many years of experience as a NICU Director in how to foster a culture of NIFCDC in a manner that provides optimal care for babies and families, while also meeting the needs of nursing staff.

LESLIE'S LEADERSHIP LIST OF 5

1. Vision
2. Infrastructure
   a. Job descriptions
   b. Competencies
   c. Policies and procedures
3. Hire the best!
   a. Interview guides
   b. Peer interviews
4. Education
   a. Competency-based orientation
   b. Neuroprotective infant and family-centered developmental care education
   c. Skills days
5. Accountability
   a. Performance reviews
   b. Peer reviews
   c. Accountability commitment sign-offs

STEP 1: HAVE A VISION FOR A CULTURE OF ACCOUNTABILITY

- Clear direction
  - Clear direction comes from unit leadership.
  - "There is no accountability in an unclear environment."
- Follow-through
  - Requires a "safe" environment, but not necessarily a "comfortable" one.
  - Focuses on goals, behaviors, and actions—just the facts.
  - Commits to dealing with behavior inconsistent with expectations.
- Rewards and consequences
  - Rewards: Simple things matter
    - Say, thank you.
    - Mention people.
    - Search for positives.
  - Consequences
    - Provide feedback and "compassionate" counseling.
    - Educate positively.
    - Assign mentors, preceptors, and coaches.

STEP 2: CREATE THE INFRASTRUCTURE BY SETTING EXPECTATIONS

- Job descriptions
  - Providing neuroprotective infant and family-centered developmental care for all patients and their families is everyone's responsibility.
    - Agree to and sign accountability commitment for:

- Service excellence
- Neuroprotective family-centered developmental care
  - Competencies
    - A neuroprotective developmentally appropriate environment for infants and families must be understood and provided.
    - Neuroprotective family-centered/integrative care skills must be learned and practiced.
  - Policies and procedures
    - Have a neuroprotective infant and family-centered developmental care policy
    - Have a family participation policy (NOT a visitation policy)
- Pay attention to the wording of policies, written documents, and in the unit signage

STEP 3: HIRE THE BEST!

- Selection criteria
  - Learn how to find the best.
  - Set high standards for selection criteria.
- Leadership interviews
  - Create an interview guide with examples of scenarios.
  - Example: Family participation at the change of shift (parents present or absent?).
- Peer interviews
  - Choose the best customer/staff-friendly nurses.
  - Create interview guides with scenarios.
  - Example: You are a new RN and not experienced with IVs. How would you handle the family's presence at the bedside of this infant?
    - Acceptable answer: I would explain that I am a rather new RN, but I have the skills for this (or I have inserted many IVs, and this is not my first time). If I am unable to get the IV in after two attempts, I will bring in another RN.
    - Acceptable answer: I would tell parents they can help support their baby during the IV procedure, or if they prefer, they could step out while I insert the IV.
    - Unacceptable answer: I would ask them to step out to the waiting room so that I can attempt the IV without someone looking over my shoulder.

STEP 4: EDUCATE AT THE BEGINNING AT ORIENTATION

- Provide competency-based orientation.
- Educate about neuroprotective infant and family-centered developmental care principles and practices.
  - Neuroprotective care needs to be built into everyone's competencies (MDs, residents, RNs, RTs, therapists, and environmental services).
  - This helps everyone to be on the same page.
  - A variety of programs can teach Neuroprotective care (eg, Wee Care, NIDCAP, etc.).

STEP 5: MAKE ACCOUNTABILITY A PRIORITY

- Continuous feedback loop
  - Provide positive feedback.

- o Provide constructive feedback and compassionate counseling.
- o Practice alternative options (role play).
- o Incorporate peer reviews.
- Accountability commitments (signed annually by each employee)
  - o Performance appraisals
  - o Service excellence statement
  - o Neuroprotective infant and family-centered developmentally appropriate care for all infants and their families

PARENT PERSPECTIVES

Lacie Dixon, RDCS, MHPS, is a family support specialist at Hand to Hold, a non-profit organization that helps to reduce the negative impact of a NICU stay and ensure the best outcome for the entire family. She has been a peer mentor with Hand to Hold since 2018. Lacie also supports NICU families at the Baylor University Medical Center - Dallas. Lacie has a Bachelor of Behavioral Science degree with a major in exercise science. She also has a specialized degree in cardiac sonography. Before joining Hand to Hold, Lacie worked in a large Children's Hospital as a registered Pediatric Cardiac Sonographer.

Lacie and her husband have two beautiful little boys, both having spent time in the NICU; Two NICU stays with two very different experiences, both with their own challenges.

Lacie's oldest son was born at 24 weeks gestational age (GA) and faced numerous hurdles throughout his 8 months in the NICU, whereas her youngest was born at 35 weeks GA.

In the early years of neonatology practice, parents were excluded from the care of their NICU babies. Fortunately, we now understand the critical importance of mothers/parents to the physiologic stability, physical growth, brain development, and emotional health of newborns and infants, no matter how prematurely they are born. Having a baby in the NICU is exceedingly stressful for parents, and rates of anxiety, postpartum depression, and post-traumatic stress disorder (PTSD) are significantly higher among NICU parents than in the general population.[6] Supporting parents during their baby's NICU stay not only benefits parents, but also supports the NICU baby's recovery, growth, and development.[7] Efforts must be consciously and sensitively made to determine the individual and changing needs of NICU parents and to provide the support they need while their baby is in the NICU. Recognizing parents as critically important to their NICU baby's well-being will lead to policies and attitudes that welcome parents to the NICU at any time, support active participation in their baby's care, and direct involvement in medical decision-making for their baby. Lacie Dixon, mother of two preterm infants, shares her NICU experience and her perspective as a parent of an ELBW baby.

LACIE'S FIRST SON'S NEONATAL INTENSIVE CARE UNIT STORY

- Gestation: 24 weeks, 0 days
- Weight: 1 lb. 9 oz
- Length: 13 inches
- Born at a local hospital with a level 3 NICU.
- Transferred at 4 weeks to Children's Hospital for patent ductus arteriosus ligation.
- Mom and dad were able to hold the baby for the first time at 7 weeks old.
- Tracheostomy and G-tube placed at 5 months. Inguinal hernia repair was performed at the same time.

- Avastin injections were given at 30 weeks due to retinopathy of prematurity diagnosis. Laser eye surgery was also required at 6 months.
- Finally, home after 8 months.

WHAT SUPPORT DO PARENTS NEED TO FEEL CONNECTED TO THEIR BABY?

- Parents need to know that they are a part of their child's care team.
- They also need to feel comfortable asking questions and helping with touch times.
- Parents in the NICU often feel like there is not much they can do for their child. This tends to make parents feel helpless, anxious, and lost in the NICU.
- It is crucial for the parents to find their place in this new environment and to know that they are an important part of the team.

WHAT SUPPORT DO PARENTS NEED TO FEEL COMFORTABLE PARTICIPATING IN THEIR BABY'S CARE?

- Parents in the NICU need patience and understanding.
- They want to participate in their baby's care, but it can be very intimidating. There is a good chance that this is the first time a parent has seen a baby this small.
- Their child is also in an incubator with numerous lines, leads, wires, and IVs.
- It is all very foreign and overwhelming.
- It takes patience from the NICU staff and a lots of hands-on learning from the parents.
- I think it is best for NICU staff to start small. Start by helping families understand what all of the wires and leads do and how to navigate them.
- Then, explain the monitors and alarms that they will hear in the NICU. The alarms alone can be triggering, so it is important to know what the sounds mean and when to worry.

WHAT WOULD PARENTS LIKE THE MEDICAL/NURSING STAFF TO KNOW ABOUT THEIR EXPERIENCE IN THE NEONATAL INTENSIVE CARE UNIT?

- While in the NICU, parents want the staff to know how overwhelmed and anxious we are.
- We want you to know that even though we have this amazing child, we are also mourning the loss of our expectations. We did not get the pregnancy or birth that we had envisioned and that is a hard pill to swallow.
- We also feel helpless, like there is nothing we can do to help our child. As a parent, it is agonizing to feel like there is little you can do when it comes to caring for your child.
- In our minds, we are supposed to be there for our little ones 24/7 and know all the right things to do and say.
- Unfortunately, this is not the case when you have a baby in the NICU, especially in a small baby unit. This realization can be heartbreaking for a parent.
- We just want to be able to hold and comfort our child. But in many cases, a parent is not able to hold their micro preemie for weeks, or in my case months.
- This goes against every instinct we have as a parent.

WHAT DOES NOT HELP SUPPORT PARENTS?

- Making the parent feel as if they are an outsider or just a "visitor" in the NICU.
- It is very hurtful to feel ignored or like our concerns are not being heard.

- Another thing that I found not helpful is starting touch times and cares early out of convenience for the staff.
- Sometimes, this is the only opportunity we have to touch or bond with our baby, and it is like a punch in the gut to show up to the NICU only to feel like these precious moments were "taken" from you.
- All of these instances can lead to feelings of inadequacy and helplessness.
- Parents want to feel like they are part of the care team, and the staff must take the extra steps to help them become more confident caregivers.

WHAT STANDS OUT TO YOU IN BEING MOST HELPFUL OR SUPPORTIVE?

- I am a big supporter and advocate for primary nurses!
- When a parent can have a team of nurses that they know and trust with their child, it makes all the difference.
- We can go home and rest with less fear and anxiety.
- Also, the NICView cameras are a wonderful resource to have, giving the parents valuable peace of mind.
- We also find that resources such as mental health professionals and peer support groups like Hand to Hold are a great asset for families.
- It is nice to know that you are not alone on this journey and others have gone through a similar experience and are on the other side of it.

WERE YOU GIVEN THE OPPORTUNITY TO BE PRESENT DURING PROCEDURES?

- Yes! Our NICU allowed parents to be present for simple procedures if they wished.
- I felt it was important to be there to console and comfort my child during these times, and it gives me comfort to think he was grateful I was there with him as well.

BABY PERSPECTIVES
Any Preterm Baby in the Neonatal Intensive Care Unit

The NICU is not the developmentally expected environment for any NICU baby, especially those born very prematurely. The sudden and unexpected transition from the womb to the NICU environment can be disorienting, disorganizing, destabilizing, and painful. Being separated from their mother is known to be incredibly stressful to all newborns and may have long-term effects.[8,9] Seeing life in the NICU from the small baby's perspective, being aware of the challenges and stressors they face, and knowing what brings them comfort and helps them cope, can motivate us to provide more consistent NIFCDC for all NICU babies. Recognizing even the smallest babies in our care as little human beings helps us recognize and appreciate their efforts at communicating with their behaviors and motivates us to treat them with dignity and respect and to respond to their needs with understanding and compassion. Here are some of the changes a small baby will experience when born too soon.

- *Womb*: warm, quiet, dim environment with continuous soft and flexible boundaries, floating in fluid, easily able to move limbs and grasp umbilical cord
  - o *NICU*: initially cold, often loud, bright environment with intermittent boundaries, on a hard surface with difficulty moving limbs against gravity and no umbilical cord to grasp
- *Womb*: encircled and contained by uterine walls and with the ability to feel the mother's movement for proprioception

○ *NICU*: often disoriented by sudden, fast movements during cares and procedures
- *Womb*: touched only by soft uterine boundaries and own hands and feet with no pain
  ○ *NICU*: touched by multiple unfamiliar hands, often roughly, often painfully
- *Womb*: continuous source of adequate nutrition and tummy full of swallowed amniotic fluid
  ○ *NICU*: often given only IV fluids with an empty stomach for several days
- *Womb*: in constant physical, hormonal, and psychological connection with mother and able to hear her familiar voice, heart rate, and body sounds
  ○ *NICU*: often separated from mother with no familiar voice and a multitude of unfamiliar sounds

SUMMARY

It takes the careful focus and collaboration of every member of the small baby team to care for the tiniest babies in the NICU. In addition to excellence in medical care, attention must be given to respectful communication, clear role definition, accountability for consistent Neuroprotective Infant and Family Centered Care practices, recognition of parents as valued members of the care team, as well as acknowledgment of the challenges extremely preterm babies face in the NICU and their urgent need for their mothers/parents for optimal healing, growth, and development.

CLINICS CARE POINTS

- Physicians and practitioners have many babies to examine and evaluate each day. Daily rounds are opportunities to be a role model for Neuroprotective Infant and Family-Centered Developmental Care (NIFCDC) and to support respectful collaboration with nurses, staff, and parents in the care of small babies.

- The scribe plays the most important role during a small baby delivery and admission. This person should have a good understanding of the goals of the golden hour and keep track of the team's progress while monitoring the infant's response to care.

- Nursing leadership can set the tone for a neonatal intensive care unit (NICU) culture of NIFCDC and, by supporting accountability, can ensure the consistency of NIFCDC practices needed to improve outcomes for ELBW infants.

- Parents are their baby's biggest advocate. No one knows their child better than its parent. Parents should be empowered to speak up and ask whatever questions they have.

- Extremely preterm babies are tiny human beings who are making a difficult and unexpected transition from womb to world. They deserve respectful and compassionate care from NICU providers and urgently need their mothers/parents for optimal stability, growth, and well-being.

ACKNOWLEDGMENTS

J. Solomon would like to give special thanks to Kathryn Fedor BSN, RNC-NIC, C-NNIC for her contributions to the quality initiative in their NICU.

DISCLOSURE

The authors have no commercial or financial conflicts of interest, no funding sources, and no disclosures to make.

REFERENCES

1. Als H, Duffy FH, McAnuity GB, et al. Early experience alters brain function and structure. Pediatrics 2004;13(4):846–57.
2. Als H, McAnulty GB. The newborn individualized developmental care and assessment program (NIDCAP) with kangaroo mother care (KMC): comprehensive care for preterm infants. Curr Womens Health Rev 2011;7(3):288–301.
3. Altimier L, Kenner C, Damus KH. The wee care neuroprotective NICU program (Wee Care): the effect of a comprehensive developmental care training program on seven neuroprotective core measures for family-centered developmental care of premature neonates. Nborn Infant Nurs Rev 2015;15:6–16.
4. Morris M, Cleary JP, Soliman A. Small baby unit improves quality and outcomes in extremely low birth weight infants. Pediatrics 2015;136:e1007–15.
5. Nankervis CA, Martin EM, Crane ML, et al. Implementation of a multidisciplinary guideline-driven approach to the care of the extremely premature infant improved hospital outcomes. Acta Paediatr 2010;99:188–93.
6. Roque ATF, Lasiuk GC, Radünz V, et al. Scoping review of the mental health of parents of infants in the NICU. J Obstet Gynecol Neonatal Nurs 2017;46(4):576–87.
7. Hynan MT, Hall SL. Psychosocial program standards for NICU parents. J Perinatol 2015;35(Suppl 1):S1–4.
8. Hofer MA. (2006). Psychobiological roots of early attachment. Curr Dir Psychol Sci 2015;15(2):84–8.
9. Leiderman PH, Seashore MJ. Mother-infant neonatal separation: some delayed consequences. Ciba Found Symp 1975;33:213–39.

Baby and Family-Centered Care in the Neonatal Intensive Care Unit: Changing Perspective

Carol B. Jaeger, DNP, RN, NNP-BC*

KEYWORDS

- Infant and family-centered care • Neurodevelopment • Developmental care • NICU
- Mother and baby closeness • Systems thinking • Epigenetics

KEY POINTS

- Providing care "with" the baby is essential rather than "to" the baby.
- Behavioral communication and the nurturing relationship of the parent(s)/family are central to managing and delivering care in the neonatal intensive care unit.
- The health care interprofessional's environment, practice, and role are to interpret the communication and guide the nurturing and interaction between the baby and parents so that the parents are integral to the baby's planning, managing, decision-making, and caregiving.
- Parents are not visitors. They are the most influential advocates and caregivers for their babies.

INTRODUCTION

Neonatal intensive care units (NICUs) have provided some form of infant and family-centered care in the United States for decades. Parents have been allowed into the NICU to visit with their baby for designated periods, and in the last decade, anytime within 24 hours per day. Some units require the parents/family to leave during shift reports and interprofessional health care team rounds. Although this practice may seem like a generous act on the part of health professionals, it robs the mother/parent(s)/family of the right to be present, informed, and to engage and connect with their baby as parents—to nurture, touch, hold, learn about their baby with their baby, perform as primary caregivers, make decisions, and *feel like a parent*.[1] As health professionals, we have spent decades learning the science of the biophysical, neurodevelopmental, and psychosocial function and communication of the baby, care methods for the

The Ohio State University, Columbus, OH, USA
* 3143 Cranston Drive, Dublin, OH 43017.
E-mail address: caroljaeger75@gmail.com

Crit Care Nurs Clin N Am 36 (2024) 185–192
https://doi.org/10.1016/j.cnc.2024.01.005
0899-5885/24/© 2024 Elsevier Inc. All rights reserved.
ccnursing.theclinics.com

baby, and outcomes; it is now time to keep the family together, and mentor the baby's parents as primary caregivers. This begins at birth.[2]

If the baby could talk, we might hear a message like this ... "I am new to this environment. My body feels different. I would rather be in the womb where I can develop with the support of nutrients and the protection of my mother. I heard voices when I was in the womb, so it is comforting to hear soft sounds. The soft voices I want to hear are those of my mother and father. They comfort and calm me. I want them near, gently touching and holding me for warmth, protection, and my mother's skin-to-skin contact for mutual regulation.[3] Please take time to understand my communication and behavior about things around me and what is happening to me in your environment and guide my parents to learn about me. Be patient so I can adapt and develop according to the ability of my mind, body, and senses. I am the best teacher of who I am, what I can do, and when I can do it."

DISCUSSION

For those NICUs integrating parent involvement before the COVID-19 pandemic, such as encouraging parents to be present as much as possible, holding their baby in skin-to-skin contact, engaging in caregiving, participating in rounds with the health care team, interacting with interprofessional quality and safety improvement opportunities and parent/family support activities, the access and involvement was severely curtailed.[4–6] Since the end of the pandemic, it has been challenging to reopen the NICU to parent inclusiveness, presence, engagement with the baby, and interaction with the health care team. The workforce[7] has been stretched as providers and staff leave employment through retirement and resignation, and others choose flexible positions and fewer work hours. Graduates begin employment with limited direct patient contact and clinical experience. Professionals in travel positions are employed with short-term contracts and need more knowledge of or commitment to unit culture and practice improvement.

Reigniting Commitment to Baby and Family-Centered Care

What can be done in the NICU to reignite the commitment to implementing baby and family-centered care, given the challenges that exist in the health care system? The connection and closeness of the baby with the mother/parents at birth is a tremendous motivator. Premature and sick babies and their parents especially need this immediate skin-to-skin intimate contact to stabilize and regulate.[8–11] Further, there is no evidence to support the practice of separating the baby and mother/parent(s).[2] Not separating them to different locations with specialty staff until the mother is discharged from inpatient care unless the health needs of the mother and baby warrant life-saving attention helps to empower parents and change the role of the interprofessional provider and caregiver so that of a guide, mentor, teacher, partner, and shared decision-maker.[2] Letting the baby and mother/parent(s) explore each other in this new nurturing environment helps the parents and health care providers/caregivers assess the biophysical and psychosocial needs of the baby and mother/parent(s).[12] We can interact with parents to learn/teach and support the parents in becoming parents—competent and confident observers, primary caregivers, innovators, and decision-makers.[13] Ask questions to help the parent verbalize the parents' engagement with and feelings toward the baby, that is, (1) what do you think the baby is telling you? (b) is the baby moving similar to the activity you felt in your womb? and (c) do some of the baby's expressions seem familiar to you? NICU, obstetric professionals, and parents can partner to assess, plan, perform, evaluate, adjust, and sustain practice together.

The separation of the baby and mother/parent immediately following birth risks increasing the stress and instability of the baby, mother, and parent.[11,14,15] They do not have the opportunity to celebrate the baby's birth together and continue as a partner in the care for the baby and mother post delivery. If separated, the mother cannot experience the care to/with the baby, and the father/parent must choose between support/presence with the baby or the mother. Neither parent has a holistic picture and understanding of the baby's care, procedures, plan, decisions, and condition. Further, the mother may be in an environment to hear the sights and sounds of healthy newborns bonding with parents/family members, which may exacerbate her feeling of failing to deliver a healthy baby.[16] Information gaps create fear and a lack of trust in the care process and health care providers and caregivers. This does not empower the parents as parents and strains the team/partner relationship that is essential for a potential long-term care process in the NICU and beyond[17,18] (**Table 1**).

Managing a medical/surgical crisis of the baby or mother is often a concern when the baby/mother/parent receives care in the same room. Communication and collaborative practice between OB and NICU caregivers can lessen anxiety. Decentralized technical communication infrastructure within NICU care spaces/rooms and personal devices carried by caregivers allow for immediate contact and response. Because the separation of the mother and baby after birth has been the way care has been delivered for decades, we do not have to perpetuate the practice. The fewer transfers and handoffs of the baby and the mother to specialty care areas/units, the less likely there will be communication errors.[19] The quality and safety of care can be improved through evidence, education and simulation learning, collaboration, and continuous improvement methods to provide a better health and well-being outcome for NICU babies and parents[20] (see **Table 1**).

Monitoring the growing relationship between the baby and parents is a continuing motivator. Keeping the baby and parent(s) together in a single-family room (SFR) can enhance the individualized learning and caregiving opportunities between the parents, providers, and staff through the in-patient NICU stay, transition to home, and continuing care at home. This collaborative partnership lessens the burden on staff and parents, strengthens the level of trust and respect, and individualizes the care of the baby and family to complement their unique culture, supportive care community, and lifestyle.

Table 1	
Benefits of non-separation and risks of separation	
Benefits of Non-separation	**Risks of Separation**
• ↓ depression in both mothers and fathers[15] • ↑ mother's breast milk production[20] • ↑ the neurologic outcomes of the baby[2] • Fewer unit transfers and handoffs[19] • Improved parent–infant attachment/bonding when together 24/7[20] • Collaborative OB/NICU provider/caregiver team care for mother and baby[19] • Co-conditioning/regulation between mother/infant/parent[23] • Immediate/early skin-to-skin contact[2,21,22] • Immediate participation in care by parents[20] • Improved observation/interpretation of infant communication and interaction[12,23,24]	• Infant stress/instability with separation of infant/mother/father[14] • Mother's emotional pain of failing to deliver a healthy baby exacerbated by a transfer to the postpartum unit surrounded by the sights/sounds of parents bonding and taking home healthy newborns[16] • Managing medical/surgical crisis events in a timely manner[20] • Ineffective communication and team collaboration between OB and NICU providers and caregivers[20,25]

If SFRs are unavailable, a comfortable space separated by a curtain or partial wall in a multi-pod room can provide privacy for baby/parent/family interaction. Reducing environmental noise in a multiuse room and in an SFR promotes baby/parent communication, voice recognition, sleep, and neurodevelopment.

Changing Perspective to the Empowerment of Parent(s)

Systems thinking, education, and simulation learning can motivate providers, staff, and parents to collaborate and innovate safe, quality care to benefit the baby and family throughout the child's lifespan.[20] Systems thinking is assessing the influence of biophysical, environmental, and psychosocial impacts on the baby/parents/family in your NICU, standardizing clinical guidelines to the evidence, and developing methods/skill sets/practices to benefit the baby and family in the short- and long-term. Learning together—providers, caregivers, parents, and family—enhances competence, collaboration, trust, and respect among each other to achieve mutual goals for the health and well-being of the baby and family. Further, collaboration among health specialties is essential to keep the biophysical, environmental, and psychosocial influences positive, practical, safe, budget-friendly, and sustaining.

The perspective of baby and family-centered care includes several process components. They are all influential in the holistic practice of baby and family-centered care. They support the management of the optimum physiologic, neurodevelopmental, and psychosocial outcomes for the baby and the family. The practice components include the following.

- Assessment of parent/family structure, socioeconomic situation, and perspective with respect for diversity, equity, and inclusivity within a just culture.[26]
- Orientation of the parent(s)/family to the birthing experience and care of the mother and baby following birth—what to expect, the role of the health care interprofessional, the role of the mother/parent(s), the opportunity to share caregiving, and decision-making.[26]
- Use systems thinking to guide/mentor the interprofessional providers and caregivers to implement parent/family presence, education, empowerment, and engagement as a primary caregiver.[26] Skin-to-skin contact enhances neurodevelopment, physiologic stability, feeding tolerance, growth, and reduced mortality and sepsis.[27]
- Use clinical guidelines to regulate baby's sleep and arousal states through baby-led communication and behavior, mother/parent contact/holding, and positioning for postural alignment, extremity movement, and physiologic stability.[28]
- Advocate and empower the role of the parent(s) as an integral member of the health interdisciplinary team and a shared decision-maker in the planning, implementation, and evaluation of care with their baby.[26]
- Continuing assessment of parent/family well-being and satisfaction intermittently during in-patient care.[29]
- The use of non-pharmacologic measures to reduce baby's stress and pain, such as immediate and continuing co-regulation with mother/parent, quiet and private environment, comfortable furnishings for parent(s) to connect/maintain closeness with their baby, reduction of procedures, as possible.[29]
- Ongoing positioning assessments of the baby's physiologic, musculoskeletal, and behavioral stability to optimize central nervous system (CNS) development and design and implement corrective measures as needed.[30]
- Facilitate behavior-based, baby-led feeding/eating, and mother/parent's competence as a primary feeder.[31]

- Transition to home with assessments of parent/family readiness, including parent competence and confidence as a caregiver and decision-maker, follow-up/continuing care plan designed and initiated, and the availability of community support to meet identified needs.[26]

Anticipated Outcomes from the Implementation of Baby and Family-Centered Care in the Neonatal Intensive Care Unit

There is a reluctance to change mindset and behavior without anticipating the outcome, especially when it involves vulnerable babies. Several published studies have provided credible evidence to frame the expectation. SFRs in the NICU are quieter, with decreased sound levels and greater temperature and humidity stability for environmental comfort.[32] A study conducted by Lester and colleagues between 2008 and 2012 compared medical and neurobehavioral outcomes at discharge in infants born less than 1500 g.[33] Participants included 151 infants in an open-bay NICU and 252 infants after transition to an SFR NICU. The infants in the SFRs exhibited the following outcomes.

- ↓ medical procedures
- ↓ time on total parenteral nutrition
- Lower gestational age at full enteral feeds
- ↓ sepsis
- ↑ sleep time
- ↑ attention
- ↓ hypertonicity
- ↓ lethargy
- ↓ pain
- ↓ physiologic stress
- ↓ LOS

Lester and colleagues concluded that the SFR is associated with improved neurobehavioral and medical outcomes. These improvements are related to increased developmental support and maternal involvement.

In the same study by Lester and colleagues, there was increased interaction by parents/family to interpret and act on signs of distress and needs of the baby, greater overall parent satisfaction, increased parent presence during the first 2 weeks of life, and positive recognition of the comfort, privacy, and environmental controls of the SFR.[33] Further, O'Callaghan and Philip reported an increase in weight on discharge, greater volume of expressed breastmilk, increased sustainment of mothers lactating and breastfeeding success, and staff satisfaction with the quality of the family and work environment in the SFR, the patient care provided, and overall job quality.[32]

Factors to consider when implementing and evaluating baby and family-centered care in SFRs of the NICU may include lower baby developmental scores if there are reduced rates of parent presence, holding skin-to-skin, and interaction between the baby and parent.[34] Further, Pineda and colleagues suggest that reduced environmental sounds may lead to lower language and motor scores on the Bayley Scales of Infant and Toddler Development at 2 years of age.[34] Another consideration is the staff's perception that providing care in NICU SFRs requires more personnel, though this concern has yet to be generally substantiated.[32] Virtual visual-audio technology in the SFRs enables NICU staff to monitor the baby when not physically present, so there has been no evidence to suggest that there is any compromise to the care of the baby. The reported metrics show decreased mortality and length of stay (LOS).[32]

SUMMARY

Given the evidence, implementation strategies, and outcomes of practicing baby and family-centered care in the NICU, why would any NICU interprofessional health professional be reticent to implement baby and family-centered care from birth to discharge? Keeping the baby close to the parents from birth is essential to the optimal outcome of the baby and the well-being of the parents and family. The challenge is to remove the system and practice barriers that impede keeping the baby and mother/parent together from birth. Innovate strategies to build, improve/maintain, and sustain the practice for the benefit of babies and families through their lifespan.

CLINICS CARE POINTS

- Change your perspective from what *you* expect … to what the *parents* expect from you.
- Connect with mother/parent(s) to learn about family structure, support person(s), socioeconomic situation, and perspective with respect for diversity, equity, and inclusivity within a just culture. Identify their expectations, fears, and concerns.
- Keep the baby and mother/parent(s) together from birth. Guide them through the process. Create a culture that values, respects, and embraces them as a family.
- Parents are members of the interprofessional health care team. Engage parents with introductions, role descriptions, and orientation to the culture and operation of the neonatal intensive care unit (NICU).
- Providers and caregivers mentor/coach parents through care, and parents teach providers and caregivers about their baby/family. Update expectations and establish mutual goals.
- Parents are essential to decision-making and care with the baby. Continually assess the collaborative relationship, the plan of care and estimated in-patient stay, improvement opportunities, family dynamics, social/economic situation, community support, questions, and concerns.
- Use parents with lived experience to provide vital information about the health care system and support to current NICU parents/families.

DISCLOSURE

The author has no commercial or financial conflicts of interest and received no funding for this article.

REFERENCES

1. Celenza JF, Zayack D, Buus-Frank ME, et al. Family involvement in quality improvement: from bedside advocate to system advisor. Clin Perinatol 2017; 44(3):553–66.
2. Bergman NJ. The neuroscience of birth–and the case for Zero Separation. Curationis 2014;37(2):e1–4.
3. Winberg J. Mother and newborn baby: mutual regulation of physiology and behavior–a selective review. Dev Psychobiol 2005;47(3):217–29.
4. Rasmussen SA, Jamieson DJ. Coronavirus disease 2019 (COVID-19) and pregnancy: responding to a rapidly evolving situation. Obstet Gynecol 2020;135(5): 999–1002.

5. Kostenzer J, Hoffmann J, von Rosenstiel-Pulver C, et al. Neonatal care during the COVID-19 pandemic - a global survey of parents' experiences regarding infant and family-centred developmental care. EClinicalMedicine 2021;39:101056.

6. Richter LL, Ku C, Mak MYY, et al. Experiences of mothers of preterm infants in the neonatal intensive care unit during the COVID-19 pandemic. Adv Neonatal Care 2023;23(4):295–303.

7. Kenner C. Neonatal nursing workforce: a global challenge and opportunity. Nborn Infant Nurs Rev 2015;15:165–6.

8. Bergman J, Bergman N. Whose choice? Advocating birthing practices according to baby's biological needs. J Perinat Educ 2013;22(1):8–13.

9. Westrup B. Newborn individualized developmental care and assessment program (NIDCAP) — family-centered developmentally supportive care. Early Hum Dev 2007;83(7):443–9.

10. Lilliesköld S, Zwedberg S, Linnér A, et al. Parents' experiences of immediate skin-to-skin contact after the birth of their very preterm neonates. J Obstet Gynecol Neonatal Nurs 2022;51(1):53–64.

11. Bry A, Wigert H. Psychosocial support for parents of extremely preterm infants in neonatal intensive care: a qualitative interview study. BMC Psychol 2019;7(1):76.

12. Rasmussen HF, Borelli JL, Smiley PA, et al. Mother-child language style matching predicts children's and mothers' emotion reactivity. Behav Brain Res 2017;325(Pt B):203–13.

13. Shaw C, Stokoe E, Gallagher K, et al. Parental involvement in neonatal critical care decision-making. Sociol Health Illness 2016;38(8):1217–42.

14. Bergman NJ. Birth practices: maternal-neonate separation as a source of toxic stress. Birth defects research 2019;111(15):1087–109.

15. Flacking R, Lehtonen L, Thomson G, et al. Closeness and separation in neonatal intensive care. Acta paediatrica (Oslo, Norway : 1992) 2012;101(10):1032–7.

16. Redshaw M, Henderson J, Bevan C. 'This is time we'll never get back': a qualitative study of mothers' experiences of care associated with neonatal death. BMJ Open 2021;11(9):e050832.

17. Stelwagen MA, van Kempen AAMW, Westmaas A, et al. Integration of maternity and neonatal care to empower parents. J Obstet Gynecol Neonatal Nurs 2020; 49(1):65–77.

18. Stelwagen M, van Kempen A, Westmaas A, et al. Parents' experiences with a model of integrated maternity and neonatal care designed to empower parents. J Obstet Gynecol Neonatal Nurs : J Obstet Gynecol Neonatal Nurs 2021;50(2): 181–92.

19. Patriksson K, Selin L. Parents and newborn "togetherness" after birth. Int J Qual Stud Health Well-Being 2022;17(1):2026281.

20. Curley A, Jones LK, Staff L. Barriers to couplet care of the infant requiring additional care: integrative review. Healthcare (Basel) 2023;11(5).

21. Crenshaw JT. Healthy birth practice #6: keep mother and baby together- it's best for mother, baby, and breastfeeding. J Perinat Educ 2014;23(4):211–7.

22. Erlandsson K, Dsilna A, Fagerberg I, et al. Skin-to-skin care with the father after cesarean birth and its effect on newborn crying and prefeeding behavior. Birth 2007;34(2):105–14.

23. Feldman R. Parent-infant synchrony and the construction of shared timing; physiological precursors, developmental outcomes, and risk conditions. J Child Psychol Psychiatry Allied Discip 2007;48(3–4):329–54.

24. Caskey M, Vohr B. Assessing language and language environment of high-risk infants and children: a new approach. Acta paediatrica (Oslo, Norway : 1992) 2013;102(5):451–61.
25. Soleimani F, Azari N, Ghiasvand H, et al. Do NICU developmental care improve cognitive and motor outcomes for preterm infants? A systematic review and meta-analysis. BMC Pediatr 2020;20(1):67.
26. Kenner C, Jaeger CB. IFCDC Recommendations for Best Practices in Systems Thinking. In: Consensus Committee of Infant and Family Centered evelopmental Care, ed. Report of the First Consensus Conference on Standards, Competencies and Best Practices for Infant and Family Centered Developmental Care in the Intensive Care Unit. https://nicudesign.nd.edu/nicu-care-standards/, 2020.
27. Phillips R, Smith K. IFCDC Recommendations for Skin-to-Skin Contact with Intimate Family Members. In: Consensus Committee of Infant and Family Centered Developmental Care, ed. Report of the First Consensus Conference on Standards, Competencies and Best Practices for Infant and Family Centered Developmental Care in the Intensive Care Unit. https://nicudesign.nd.edu/nicu-care-standards/, 2020.
28. Bigsby R, Salisbury A. IFCDC Recommendations for Best Practices to Support Sleep and Arousal. In: Consensus Committee of Infant and Family Centered Developmental Care, ed. Report of the First Consensus Conference on Standards, Competencies and Best Practices for Infant and Family Centered Developmental Care in the Intensive Care Unit. https://nicudesign.nd.edu/nicu-care-standards/, 2020.
29. Hynan M, Cicco R, Hatfield B. IFCDC Recommendations for Best Practice Reducing and Managing Pain and Stress in Newborns and Families. In: Consensus Committee of Infant and Family Centered Developmental Care, ed. Report of the First Consensus Conference on Standards, Competencies and Best Practices for Infant and Family Centered Developmental Care in the Intensive Care Unit. https://nicudesign.nd.edu/nicu-care-standards/, 2020.
30. Sweeney J, McElroy J. IFCDC Recommendations for Best Practice for Positioning and Touch. In: Consensus Committee of Infant and Family Centered Developmental Care, ed. Report of the First Consensus Committee on Standards, Competencies and Best Practices for Infant and Family Centered Developmental Care in the Intensive Care Unit. https://nicudesign.nd.edu/nicu-care-standards/, 2020.
31. Ross E, Arvedson JC, McGrath J. IFCDC Recommendations for Best Practices for Feeding, Eating and Nutrition Delivery. In: Consensus Committee of Infant and Family Developmental Care, ed. Report of the First Consensus Conference on Standards, Competencies and Best Practices for Infant and Family Centered Developmental Care in the Intensive Care Unit. https://nicudesign.nd.edu/nicu-care-standards/, 2020.
32. O'Callaghan N, Dee A, Philip RK. Evidence-based design for neonatal units: a systematic review. Matern Health Neonatol Perinatol 2019;5:6.
33. Lester BM, Hawes K, Abar B, et al. Single-family room care and neurobehavioral and medical outcomes in preterm infants. Pediatrics 2014;134(4):754–60.
34. Pineda RG, Stransky KE, Rogers C, et al. The single-patient room in the NICU: maternal and family effects. J Perinatol 2012;32(7):545–51.

Pain in Neonates
Perceptions and Current Practices

Marsha Campbell-Yeo, PhD, MN, NNP-BC, RN[a,b,*],
Morgan MacNeil, BScN, RN[a,b,1], Helen McCord, BScN, RN, MN, NNP[a,b,2]

KEYWORDS

- Neonate • Infant • Pain • Assessment • Management • Parent perceptions

KEY POINTS

- All newborn infants experience pain as a part of routine care. Repeated exposure to untreated pain in premature infants has been linked with long-lasting negative effects.
- Despite the significant adverse effects associated with untreated pain in infants, combined with the availability of effective methods to prevent and reduce pain, most infants will receive ineffective or no treatment.
- Despite the compelling evidence that we have to guide infant pain assessment and management, significant knowledge gaps exist among parents, nurses, and other health-care providers.
- The subjective and complex nature of pain, especially when present in a nonverbal population, poses a significant challenge in pain assessment for health-care providers.
- Effective pain management is a standard of care for all infants in the neonatal intensive care unit. The most effective method to eliminate infant pain is to reduce the number of procedures performed.

INTRODUCTION

All newborn infants experience pain as a part of routine care, such as vitamin K injections and heel pokes to obtain blood for screening tests, within the first hours and days following birth.[1–3] Most will undergo up to 20 injections to prevent diseases in their first 2 years.[4] In healthy newborns, exposure to pain in early life has been associated with physiologic instability, greater inflammatory reaction, and hypersensitivity to subsequent pain.[5,6] Data from 18 epidemiologic studies from numerous countries examining

[a] Faculty of Health, School of Nursing, Dalhousie University, Halifax, Nova Scotia, Canada;
[b] MOM-LINC Lab, IWK Health, Halifax, Nova Scotia, Canada
[1] Present address: 820 Monte Vista Road, Enfield, Nova Scotia B2T 1H9, Canada.
[2] Present address: 41 Sheltered Lane, Upper Tantallon, Nova Scotia B3Z 0H2, Canada.
* Corresponding author. MOM-LINC Lab, IWK Health, 5850/5980 University Avenue, Halifax, Nova Scotia, B3K 6R8, Canada.
E-mail address: marsha.campbell-yeo@dal.ca
Twitter: @DrMCampbellYeo (M.C.-Y.); @morganxmacneil (M.M.)

Crit Care Nurs Clin N Am 36 (2024) 193–210
https://doi.org/10.1016/j.cnc.2023.11.004
0899-5885/24/© 2023 Elsevier Inc. All rights reserved.

the frequency of exposure to painful procedures in premature infants in a neonatal intensive care unit (NICU), demonstrated that infants undergo 7 to 17 procedures daily.[7]

Repeated exposure to untreated pain in premature infants has been linked with changes in hemodynamics and increased intracranial pressure.[8,9] In addition to these immediate adverse effects, repeated pain exposure has been associated with multiple long-lasting effects impacting future pain processing, vision, ability to learn, control emotions, behaviors, and movement.[5,6] The number of exposures to untreated pain in infants born very prematurely, controlling for gestational age at birth and comorbidities, have been linked to overall brain growth, including reduced thalamic and cerebellar growth, frontal and partial brain width and alteration in gray–white matter ratios, and temporal lobe functional connectivity.[5,6,10–13] Changes in expected epigenetic programming and telomere growth have also been reported.[14,15]

Despite the significant adverse effects associated with untreated pain in infants, combined with the availability of effective methods to prevent and reduce pain, most infants will receive ineffective or no treatment.[7,16]

PARENT HEALTH-CARE PROVIDER PERCEPTIONS

Parents are an essential component of the comprehensive assessment and management of infant pain, through reading infant pain cues and using interventions such as breastfeeding and skin-to-skin contact (SSC). However, the utilization of parent-led interventions is reliant on parental knowledge and perceptions about pain and how pain is managed during hospitalization.[17] Parents, namely mothers, report a strong desire to be involved in pain management practices for their infant. Despite this desire, mothers report that they feel underutilized by health-care providers in the provision of pain management for their infants, which leaves mothers feeling helpless as their infants experience pain.[18] It is the responsibility of the health-care provider to educate parents on how they can be involved with managing infant pain and provide them with guidance during painful procedures.

In a study examining parental knowledge surrounding infant pain management, only 61.4% of mothers and 30.4% of fathers thought that they could reduce their infant's pain. Furthermore, only 40.3% of mothers and 26.1% of fathers reported that interventions such as breastfeeding were useful in reducing an infant's pain.[19] This study confirms that a substantial knowledge gap exists among parents surrounding effective parent-led infant pain management.

Nurses play an integral role in pain assessment and management in infant populations. Their clinical judgment, decision-making, and collaboration with other members of the multidisciplinary team pave the way for optimal infant pain assessment and management.[20–22] Despite the available evidence-based resources for nurses to guide pain assessment and management in this vulnerable population, various matters can affect how nurses assess and subsequently manage pain in infants, including knowledge, attitudes, clinical outcomes, communication issues, and fear of side effects from pharmacologic interventions.[20,23]

A systematic review investigating nurses' and midwives' knowledge in assessing and managing infant pain in the NICU context described a low level of clinical knowledge of infant pain, serving as an explanation for the lack of adequate pain management interventions.[23] Some studies retrieved from this systematic review revealed that nurses rarely use a formal pain assessment tool to guide their analysis of infant pain and instead rely on their own knowledge and experience.[23–26] Nurses working in the clinical setting have varying years of experience, educational backgrounds, and personal experiences so the lack of reliance on evidence-based pain assessment tools to guide infant pain assessment is concerning.

A study examining pain management knowledge among NICU health-care providers revealed that nurses and neonatologists demonstrated a lack of knowledge surrounding the use of opioids for pain management because they opted to use sedation medications (eg, chloral hydrate) in place of opioids. Moreover, this study concluded that neonatal nurses preferred to use nonpharmacological interventions to manage infant pain in comparison to neonatologists.[27] This discrepancy between the viewpoints of neonatal nurses and neonatologists regarding effective infant pain management supports the need for additional education among NICU health-care providers.

Findings from these studies demonstrate that despite the compelling evidence that we have to guide infant pain assessment and management, significant knowledge gaps exist among parents, nurses, and other health-care providers.

PAIN ASSESSMENT

Numerous national and international level guidelines focused on infant pain management state that pain assessment is integral to evaluating the need for, as well as the efficacy of, pain-relieving interventions across different situations.[28–30] Basing pain management interventions on a comprehensive pain assessment prevents infants from being undertreated or overtreated.

Self-report is the gold-standard method of pain assessment in adult populations and cognitively intact persons.[31] However, in nonverbal populations, such as infants, health-care providers must rely on alternative assessment methods to assist in painting a comprehensive picture of the pain experienced and subsequently achieve optimal pain management. The subjective and complex nature of pain, especially when present in a nonverbal population, poses a significant challenge in pain assessment for health-care providers.[31]

Indicators of infant pain are commonly categorized into behavioral, physiologic, hormonal, or neurophysiological domains (**Table 1** adapted from Campbell-Yeo and colleagues).[31,32] It is well understood that pain is highly subjective and multidimensional. Thus, a multidimensional approach to pain assessment that is validated to detect all painful situations (high sensitivity), distinguish noxious from nonnoxious stimuli (high specificity), measure the type of pain that clinicians are aiming to measure (validity), yield consistent results when used between clinicians (reliability), and establish whether pain management interventions were effective or not (responsiveness), is recommended.[32,33] Most commonly used pain assessment tools can be found in **Table 2**.

PAIN MANAGEMENT

Effective pain management, which can improve clinical and neurodevelopmental outcomes, is a standard of care for all infants in the NICU.[32,57] The most effective method to eliminate infant pain is to reduce the number of procedures performed.[58] Infant pain management interventions can be categorized as nonpharmacologic, sweet-tasting, and pharmacologic.

Nonpharmacologic Interventions

Nonpharmacologic interventions are recommended as the first-line treatment of pain in infants. These interventions can reduce pain while also providing comfort and minimizing stress.[59,60] Multiple nonpharmacologic strategies can be used simultaneously to provide optimal pain management to infants.[61] Many of these interventions are

Table 1
Infant pain indicators

Indicator Domain	Description
Behavioral	
Alertness and sleep–wake state	• Hyperalert states are seen when pain is ongoing or prolonged • Younger or sicker infants may require longer time to comfort themselves and return to a resting state after exposure to a painful stimulus
Body movements	• Preterm infants often display diffuse movements that are harder to control • Younger or sicker infants can turn flaccid, as opposed to strong infants who react with increased muscle tension in the extremities
Crying	• Healthy, awake, full-term infants may display crying that becomes more intense and prolonged with increasing discomfort • Lower gestational age, sick, sleeping, or sedated infants may not have a vocal reaction

Facial expressions	• Common facial expressions linked to pain:
	  ○ Brow bulge
	  ○ Eye squeeze
	  ○ Distinct furrows from the nose to the ends of the mouth
	  ○ Tense and stretched mouth/tongue
	  ○ Raised cheeks

Physiologic	
Heart rate and heart rate variability	• Healthy, full-term infants often show increased heart rate, blood pressure, and erythema • Younger, sicker infants may have fluctuations in heart rate • Pain reduces heart rate variability over time; therefore, heart rate variability is best suited for the assessment of prolonged pain exposure
Respiratory rate	• In healthy, full-term infants, respirations will increase in the presence of pain. In preterm infants, respirations decrease or are even absent (apnea) due to pain exposure • When pain is present in the thorax region of the body, it may lead to breathing difficulty or cessation
Oxygen saturation	• Oxygen saturation changes follow pain-associated changes in respiration and heart rate • Increases or decreases can be observed (context dependent)
Cortisol	• Increased levels are common after surgery[34] and painful procedures[35]
Neurophysiological	
Cerebral oxygenation	• Measured using near-infrared spectroscopy associated with cerebral activation and changes in oxygenated and deoxygenated levels of hemoglobin in the brain • High levels of oxygenated hemoglobin may reflect neuronal activation caused by pain

(continued on next page)

Table 1 (continued)	
Indicator Domain	**Description**
Electroencephalogram (EEG) and evoked potentials	• Multichannel EEG used as a proxy for neuronal activity with numerous studies reporting on pain-related event-related potentials during pain exposure[36,37]
Functional MRI	• Has the ability to show which areas of an infant's brain are activated when exposed to pain[38]

cost-effective, easy to implement into everyday nursing practice, and are associated with little to no risk.[62]

Breastfeeding

Multiple studies have confirmed breastfeeding as one of the most effective interventions in relieving pain for infants undergoing painful procedures.[63,64] The mechanisms involved in breastfeeding (i.e., holding, SSC, suckling, distracting, and ingesting breastmilk) work together to provide pain relief to infants. Studies have concluded that breastfeeding effectively reduces pain-related behavioral and physiologic responses, as well as pain scores when compared with positioning, mother holding, placebo, or no intervention.[64,65] Moreover, it has been shown that while expressed breastmilk alone without maternal contact provides some pain relief when compared with no treatment, it remains less effective than direct breastfeeding or sucrose administration.[60,64] Despite the numerous benefits associated with breastfeeding, it is not a viable option for all infants cared for in the NICU, such as very preterm infants or those who are intubated and ventilated.[66]

Skin-to-skin contact

SSC occurs when a naked infant (with or without a diaper) is held in an upright position on a family member's bare chest. A Cochrane systematic review on SSC for the

Table 2 Infant pain assessment tools	
Pain Type	**Assessment Scale Name**
Acute procedural pain	ABC[39]
	BIIP[40]
	BPSN[41,42]
	Douleur Aigue Nouveau-ne[43]
	Faceless Acute Neonatal Pain Scale[44]
	Face, Legs, Activity, Cry, Consolability scale[45]
	Neonatal Facial Coding System[46]
	Neonatal Infant Pain Scale[47]
	Neonatal Infant Acute Pain Assessment Scale[48]
	Premature Infant Pain Profile—Revised (PIPP, PIPP-R)[49,50]
Postoperative pain	Neonatal Pain, Agitation and Sedation Scale[51]
	Pain Assessment Tool[52]
Prolonged pain	Astrid Lindgren and Lund Children's Hospital's Pain and Stress Assessment Scale for Preterm and Sick Newborn Infants[53]
	COMFORT[54]
	Échelle Douleur inconfort Nouveau-né[55]
	Multidimensional Assessment of Pain Scale[56]

Abbreviations: BIIP, behavioral indicators of infant pain; BPSN, bernese pain scale for neonates.

management of procedural pain reported that SSC was effective in reducing infant pain for a single procedure such as a heel stick.[67] SSC provides the same pain-reducing efficacy as sucrose.[31,68]

Most studies examining the effects of SSC focus only on mothers. However, health-care providers should also encourage fathers and other family members to engage in SSC and other pain management practices with the infant because there is some evidence to suggest that they are equally as effective as mothers.[69] Nurses play a vital role in facilitating SSC for minor painful procedures because these can be scheduled in partnership with families. Health-care providers should aim to prioritize the utilization of parent-led strategies to optimize parental involvement in their infants' care.[70]

Nonnutritive sucking

Nonnutritive sucking (NNS) is the placement of a pacifier, gloved finger, or infant's digit in the mouth to promote sucking in the absence of a feed.[71] A Cochrane systematic review demonstrated that NNS improved regulation after painful procedures in both preterm and full-term infants.[72] Although not an optimal sole intervention, NNS is an effective pain-reduction adjuvant strategy in infants undergoing acute procedural pain,[31,60] and has been reported that NNS used in conjunction with sucrose is more effective than NNS used alone.[73] Breastfeeding and oral sucrose combined with NNS remain the preferred methods for pain from minor painful procedures in full-term healthy infants.[28]

Swaddling/facilitated tucking

Swaddling is a simple and safe technique that can also be used as an adjuvant strategy in combination with other pain-reducing interventions by nurses and families to help reduce minor procedural pain in infants.[74] Swaddling involves gently wrapping an infant in a blanket while keeping the infant's limbs flexed, which facilitates self-soothing behaviors.[42] Facilitated tucking has also been described as a physical containment method that nests the infant, bringing the body to midline by holding the upper and lower extremities of the infant in flexion with hands rather than a blanket.[75] Both swaddling and facilitated tucking are easy to do, cost-effective, and developmentally supportive. Swaddling and facilitated tucking are more effective than no intervention in reducing pain in minor painful procedures in term[60,76] and preterm infants[77]; however, they are most effective when used in combination with other interventions such as sucrose.[78]

Sweet tasting solutions

Breastfeeding and SSC are considered first-line therapies for infant pain, with sweet-tasting solutions as an alternative if a parent is unavailable. Oral sucrose is a widely studied treatment for the management of infant procedural pain.[78-81] Both oral sucrose and glucose have been reported to reduce procedural pain in preterm and term infants.[78,82] These sweet-tasting agents are hypothesized to work via the activation of the endogenous opioid system; however, the exact mechanism of action remains unclear.[78] Although sucrose used alone is effective, there is evidence to support that sucrose used in combination with NNS may add additional benefits.[68,83] Although evidence related to optimal sucrose dosing is limited, data suggest that volumes as low as 0.1 mL and repeated throughout the painful procedure are effective.[84] Additional research is required to confirm the efficacy of sucrose used in extremely preterm infants, as well as the impact of sucrose on neurodevelopmental outcomes.

Pharmacologic Interventions

Pharmacologic interventions are the most frequently used methods of pain management for major procedures and surgical interventions in the NICU.[81] There are existing knowledge gaps related to the optimal use of pharmacologic interventions to manage pain in infants, such as a lack of data on efficacy and uncertainty regarding possible adverse effects of long-term neurodevelopmental outcomes.[31] Despite the need for ongoing research to help address these gaps, the known adverse effects of untreated pain in infants have led to the consistent inclusion of pharmacologic interventions in pain management guidelines for infants.[31,85]

Opioids

Opioids are known to provide analgesia across all age groups, and administration of opioids is the first choice for the management of surgical or major painful procedures in the NICU.[86] The most widely used opioids in NICUs include morphine and fentanyl. Due to the potential risk of associated adverse effects (i.e., respiratory depression, hypotension, and urinary retention), safe and effective dosing to achieve the optimal balance between effective pain management and opioid overuse, especially in infants born extremely preterm and infants requiring prolonged ventilation, remains a challenge.[31,87] A recent Cochrane review examined the effects and safety of pharmacologic interventions related to pain and sedation management to prevent germinal matrix hemorrhage and intraventricular hemorrhage (GMH-IVH) in ventilated preterm infants.[88] This study demonstrated that opioids have no or less effect on GMH-IVH (any grade), severe intraventricular hemorrhage, all-cause infant death, or major neurodevelopmental disability.[88]

A study assessing the benefits and harms of opioids in preterm and term infants undergoing a painful procedure found that when compared with a placebo, there is moderate evidence that opioids reduce procedural pain assessed using pain scales during the procedure; however, it may not make a difference with other scales 1 to 2 hours after the procedure.[86] The evidence was deemed uncertain about the effect of opioids when compared with nonpharmacologic measures or other analgesics for some procedures.[86] Although uncertain evidence demonstrates that continuous intravenous infusions provide more effective pain management with fewer adverse effects than intermittent bolus, more research is warranted to inform a consensus recommendation.[60,89]

Nonopioid analgesics

Acetaminophen. Acetaminophen is one of the most used analgesic medications in NICU, despite the lack of evidence to support effective pain relief in infants undergoing acute painful procedures.[90]

Nonsteroidal anti-inflammatory drugs. The use of nonsteroidal anti-inflammatory drugs (NSAIDs; eg, ibuprofen, ketorolac, ketoprofen, and indomethacin) that are commonly used among older children is less common in the infant population given the increased risk for renal injury and gastrointestinal bleeding.[91] In fact, most NSAIDs are not approved for usage in infants less than 6 months of age.[31,91,92] The populations at highest risk for negative outcomes in association with NSAID exposure include infants less than 3 weeks of age and those delivered prematurely.[91] Due to the substantial risks, no recommendations can be made regarding the use of NSAIDs for procedural pain relief.[31]

N-methyl-D-aspartate receptor antagonists. The N-methyl-D-aspartate (NMDA) receptor is a receptor of glutamate, the primary excitatory neurotransmitter in the human brain. NMDA receptor antagonists, such as ketamine, provide a sedative, analgesic, and amnesic effect.[93] Research on NMDA receptor antagonists is limited due to concern over their side effects, limiting clinical application. A Cochrane review concluded that the evidence is very uncertain about the effect of ketamine on pain scores during painful procedures compared with placebo or fentanyl.[94] Therefore, no recommendations can be made regarding the use of NMDA receptor antagonists for procedural pain relief, and further research is required before formal recommendations can be made for administration in this population.[94]

Dexmedetomidine. Intravenous dexmedetomidine has been shown that it may be an effective agent for pain treatment and sedation in infants.[95] Dexmedetomidine is an alpha-2 adrenergic receptor agonist that produces sedation and analgesia and may be associated with fewer serious side effects such as respiratory depression.[96] A small animal study demonstrated that dexmedetomidine may also play a neuroprotective role.[62] Unfortunately, no studies have been conducted to determine the long-term neurologic outcomes of the use of dexmedetomidine in the neonatal period, which remains a considerable concern for health-care providers.[95]

Topical Anesthetics

A Cochrane review concluded that there was not enough quality evidence to determine if topical anesthetics can help relieve needle-related pain in newborns in the first month after birth.[97] Eutectic mixture of local anesthetics, which is a combination of 2.5% prilocaine and 2.5% lidocaine, was not shown to reduce pain associated with heel lancing[98] but may reduce pain associated with lumbar puncture needle insertions.[97] Evidence confirms that topical anesthetics used alone are insufficient in providing pain relief.[99] Caution is warranted when using topical anesthetics in extremely preterm infants because there is a dearth of evidence to support their efficacy and safety.

Evidence supports the use of topical anesthetic eye drops during routine eye examinations for retinopathy of prematurity (ROP) screening.[100] To date, no intervention has been found to provide an effective reduction in the moderate-to-severe pain associated with eye examinations. Current evidence demonstrates the use of a multi-intervention approach that includes the use of topical eye drops in conjunction with 24% sucrose (or equivalent glucose solution) NNS, swaddling/containment, and parent voice, when possible, to achieve optimal pain management.[31,101] Further research is warranted to explore alternatives and more effective interventions are needed.

Sedatives

Sedatives are used to alter the level of consciousness in a patient and are commonly used as adjuncts to analgesics.[102] Commonly used sedatives in the NICU include benzodiazepines, barbiturates, choral hydrate, and dexmedetomidine. Due to the lack of evidence to support the efficacy and safety associated with the use of sedatives in preterm and term populations, they are not used routinely in the NICU setting.[60] Of major concern is the fact that sedatives do not provide significant analgesia while altering the infant's level of consciousness and, therefore, may hide the clinical signs of pain.[60,103] Midazolam is contraindicated for infants less than 34 weeks, due to the elevated risk associated with hypotension and neurologic injury.[104] Therefore, sedatives should be used with extreme caution and never alone as a sole agent for infant pain.[102]

GAPS AND FUTURE RESEARCH DIRECTIONS

Although significant strides have been made in the world of infant pain assessment and management, there remains a paucity of evidence surrounding the pain care of vulnerable populations, namely, infants with and at risk for intellectual disabilities, infants with ROP, infants diagnosed with neonatal abstinence syndrome, and extremely low birth weight infants. Moreover, there remains a need for further research on additional pain-relieving interventions, such as cooling therapy.

Infants with and at Risk for Intellectual Disabilities

Infants with intellectual disabilities, characterized by significant limitations in intellectual functioning and adaptive behavior, and those infants at risk for developing intellectual disabilities are at an increased risk of ubiquitous pain exposure.[105,106] This increased risk is largely due to the etiologic nature of intellectual disabilities, which may affect numerous bodily systems and processes, leading to the need for invasive diagnostic tests and procedures, such as recurrent bloodwork.[107–109]

Despite the global investment in pediatric pain during the past 3 decades, researchers and clinicians know very less about how infants with and at risk for intellectual disabilities perceive, process, and respond to pain. This paucity of knowledge increases these already highly vulnerable infants' risk for developing negative health outcomes because of mismanaged pain, diagnostic overshadowing, and stigmatization.[106,110]

Retinopathy of Prematurity

Screening eye examinations for ROP is standard practice across NICUs globally. ROP is one of the leading causes of preventable blindness in children and is unique to premature infants.[111] ROP originates from the immature vasculature that is present in a preterm infant's retina.[112] In Canada, it is recommended that all infants born 30 6/7 weeks' gestational age or lesser and infants having a birth weight 1250 g or lesser are screened for ROP.[112] These criteria lead to a significant number of screened infants who are experiencing considerable pain and distress associated with the examination.[112,113] Although various interventions have been implemented in practice to reduce the amount of pain experienced by these infants, no single intervention has been proven effective.

Topical anesthetic eye drops and oral sucrose are used most frequently to manage pain in ROP eye examinations, despite evidence showing minimal to no pain-relieving effect when using these agents alone.[60,78,114] Topical anesthetic eye drops can help to reduce pain; however, when used as a single agent, they do not provide optimal pain relief.[100] One study suggested intranasal fentanyl was more effective than intranasal saline in reducing pain associated with ROP screening; however, additional evidence is required.[115] There remains a vital need to identify effective interventions for standard pain relief measures undertaken during ROP screening.

Neonatal Abstinence Syndrome

Another population with a paucity of information regarding the effective assessment and management of pain are infants diagnosed with neonatal abstinence syndrome (NAS) more recently referred to as neonatal opioid withdrawal syndrome (NOWS).[116] NOWS originates from prenatal exposure to opioid substances such as morphine or methadone and is generally manifested as a group of symptoms including central nervous system disturbances such as seizures, tremors, and excessive crying, alterations in metabolic, vasomotor, and respiratory systems exhibited by sweating or tachypnea, or gastrointestinal upset including poor feeding or vomiting.[116] Given the cascade of these symptoms, these infants have typically been excluded from studies examining pain assessment or the effectiveness of interventions to reduce pain associated with procedures. As such, less information is known regarding the

Table 3
Practice recommendations for infant pain care

Institution	Health-care facilities providing care to newborns should establish an organization-wide pain management framework with dedicated resources that includes comprehensive training for care providers and implementation and quality improvement strategies to ensure optimal prevention and management of pain
Prevention	All efforts should be taken to minimize bloodwork and procedures. Noninvasive monitoring should be used when possible and prescribers should justify that the benefits of conducting the procedure outweigh potential harms
Assessment	All care providers should receive and have access to training to assess newborns for pain using gestational age appropriate and valid multidimensional tools
	Pain assessment should be performed regularly, recorded and reported, following an algorithm with specified actions for each level of pain to guide care
	Pain assessments should be conducted at least once per shift, more frequently if the infant is receiving pain reducing medications and following adjustments in pain management interventions to evaluate effectiveness and determine possible need for additional intervention
	Parents should be actively engaged in pain assessment and management
Management	Parent led interventions such as direct breastfeeding or SSC should be considered as a first-line pain management for needle-related procedures
	Sweet tasting solutions combined with NNS should be considered as a second-line management, if it is not possible to coordinate to have a parent present
	Use of other types of nonpharmacologic interventions as adjuvant therapies should be considered
	Topical anesthetic eye drops in combination with a sweet tasting solution, NNS, containment, and parent presence or voice should be provided during eye examinations for the screening of ROP
	Topical anesthetic provided before a lumbar puncture at the time of needle insertion should be considered, although smaller doses may be required and used with caution in extremely preterm infants
	Topical anesthetic should be used in combination with a regional anesthetic during circumcision
	Acetaminophen/paracetamol should not routinely be used for treatment of procedural pain
	Acetaminophen/paracetamol should be considered postoperatively as an adjuvant therapy
	All infants undergoing nonemergent endotracheal intubation, including brief or noninvasive surfactant administration, should receive effective analgesic
	Use of opioids during invasive mechanical ventilation should be used based on the evaluation of valid pain assessment tools
	Opioids should be used to reduce pain associated with major invasive procedures (eg, chest tube insertion) and postoperatively
	Continuous infusion versus intermittent bolus of opioids should be considered for longer lasting procedures or postoperatively
	Sedative agents should be used with caution and if used should be considered as an adjuvant therapy and not be provided alone as a sole agent. Midazolam is contraindicated for infants <34 weeks

most effective ways to manage pain in this group of infants, and future research is warranted.

Extremely Low Birth Weight

Infants born extremely preterm, between 22 and 25 weeks, have been significantly underrepresented in infant pain studies. These infants usually have high acuity and exposure to repeated pain. Moreover, given the extreme underdevelopment of their brain, they are at the highest risk for short-term and long-term adverse outcomes associated with untreated pain.[117,118] Future studies are warranted to determine optimal pain management.

COOLING THERAPY

Many questions remain regarding optimal pain care during hypothermic whole-body or head cooling for infants at risk for hypoxic-ischemic encephalopathy. In a review of 10 studies (1 randomized controlled trial and 9 observational with serious risk of bias) including 2551 infants reporting on the optimal management of pain and stress for infants undergoing therapeutic hypothermia for hypoxic-ischemic encephalopathy, the authors stated that given the paucity and very low certainty evidence, no recommendations could be determined.[119] Similarly, in a 2022 Cochrane review examining pharmacologic interventions for pain and sedation management in newborn infants undergoing therapeutic hypothermia, no randomized clinical studies meeting eligibility criteria were found.[120]

IMPLICATIONS FOR PRACTICE

Considering the quality of the existing evidence, the practice recommendations found in **Table 3** should be used to guide institutional and individual health-care provider practice.

CLINICS CARE POINTS

- Health-care facilities providing care to newborns should establish an organization-wide pain management framework with dedicated resources that include comprehensive training for care providers and implementation and quality improvement strategies to ensure optimal prevention and management of pain.

- All efforts should be taken to minimize bloodwork and procedures. Noninvasive monitoring should be used when possible and prescribers should justify that the benefits of conducting the procedure outweigh potential harms.

- All care providers should receive and have access to training to assess newborns for pain using gestational age-appropriate and valid multidimensional tools. Pain assessment should be performed regularly, recorded, and reported, following an algorithm with specified actions for each level of pain to guide care.

- Parent-led interventions such as direct breastfeeding or SSC should be considered as first-line pain management for needle-related procedures, and sweet-tasting solutions combined with NNS should be considered as second-line management if it is not possible to coordinate having a parent present.

DISCLOSURE

The authors have nothing to disclose.

REFERENCES

1. Puckett RM, Offringa M. Prophylactic vitamin K for vitamin K deficiency bleeding in neonates. Cochrane Database Syst Rev 2000. https://doi.org/10.1002/14651858. CD002776.
2. Ng E, Loewy AD. Guidelines for vitamin K prophylaxis in newborns. Paediatr Child Health 2018;23(6):394–7.
3. Therrell BL, Padilla CD, Loeber JG, et al. Current status of newborn screening worldwide: 2015. Semin Perinatol 2015;39(3):171–87.
4. Centers for Disease Control and Prevention (CDC). Birth-18 Years Immunization Schedule. https://www.cdc.gov/vaccines/schedules/hcp/imz/child-adolescent. html.
5. Vinall J, Grunau RE. Impact of repeated procedural pain-related stress in infants born very preterm. Pediatr Res 2014;75(5):584–7.
6. Walker SM. Long-term effects of neonatal pain. Semin Fetal Neonatal Med 2019; 24(4):101005.
7. Cruz MD, Fernandes AM, Oliveira CR. Epidemiology of painful procedures performed in neonates: a systematic review of observational studies. Eur J Pain 2016;20(4):489–98.
8. Mcgrath PJ, Latimer M, Finley A, et al. Measurement of pain in children, 14, 2009.
9. Craig KD, Whitfield MF, Grunau RVE, et al. Pain in the preterm neonate: behavioural and physiological indices. Pain 1993;52(3):287–99.
10. Ranger M, Zwicker JG, Chau CMY, et al. Neonatal pain and infection relate to smaller cerebellum in very preterm children at school age. J Pediatr 2015; 167(2):292–8.e1.
11. Duerden EG, Grunau RE, Guo T, et al. Early procedural pain is associated with regionally-specific alterations in thalamic development in preterm neonates. J Neurosci 2018;38(4):878–86.
12. Brummelte S, Grunau RE, Chau V, et al. Procedural pain and brain development in premature newborns. Ann Neurol 2012;71(3):385–96.
13. Doesburg SM, Chau CM, Cheung TPL, et al. Neonatal pain-related stress, functional cortical activity and visual-perceptual abilities in school-age children born at extremely low gestational age. Pain 2013;154(10):1946–52.
14. Chau CMY, Ranger M, Sulistyoningrum D, et al. Neonatal pain and COMT Val158Met genotype in relation to serotonin transporter (SLC6A4) promoter methylation in very preterm children at school age. Front Behav Neurosci 2014;8. https://doi.org/10.3389/fnbeh.2014.00409.
15. Provenzi L, Giusti L, Fumagalli M, et al. Pain-related stress in the Neonatal Intensive Care Unit and salivary cortisol reactivity to socio-emotional stress in 3-month-old very preterm infants. Psychoneuroendocrinology 2016;72:161–5.
16. Orovec A, Disher T, Caddell K, et al. Assessment and management of procedural pain during the entire neonatal intensive care unit hospitalization. Pain Manag Nurs 2019;20(5):503–11.
17. Franck LS, Oulton K, Bruce E. Parental involvement in neonatal pain management: an empirical and conceptual update. J Nurs Scholarsh 2012;44(1):45–54.
18. Kyololo OM, Stevens BJ, Songok J. Mothers' perceptions about pain in hospitalized newborn infants in Kenya. J Pediatr Nurs 2019;47:51–7.
19. Vazquez V, Cong X, DeJong A. Maternal and paternal knowledge and perceptions regarding infant pain in the NICU. Neonatal Network 2015;34(6):337–44.

20. Andersen RD, Nakstad B, Jylli L, et al. The complexities of nurses' pain assessment in hospitalized preverbal children. Pain Manag Nurs 2019;20(4):337–44.

21. Association of Women's Health O and NN. Neonatal nursing: clinical competencies and education guide, 7th edition. Nurs Womens Health 2019;23(3): e23–35.

22. Skorobogatova N, Žemaitienė N, Šmigelskas K, et al. Limits of professional competency in nurses working in NICU. Open Med 2018;13(1):410–5.

23. Mala O, Forster EM, Kain VJ. Neonatal nurse and midwife competence regarding pain management in neonates. Adv Neonatal Care 2022;22(2):E34–42.

24. Cong X, McGrath JM, Delaney C, et al. Neonatal nurses' perceptions of pain management: survey of the United States and China. Pain Manag Nurs 2014; 15(4):834–44.

25. Barros MMA, Luiz BVS, Mathias CV. Pain as the fifth vital sign: nurse's practices and challenges in a neonatal intensive unit care. Brazilian Journal Of Pain 2019; 2(3). https://doi.org/10.5935/2595-0118.20190041.

26. Mehrnoush N, Ashktorab T, heidarzadeh M, et al. Pain management perceptions of the neonatal nurses in NICUS and neonatal units in Ardebil, Iran. Iranian Journal of Neonatology 2016;7(4):23–9.

27. Peng NH, Lee MC, Su WL, et al. Knowledge, attitudes, and practices of neonatal professionals regarding pain management. Eur J Pediatr 2021;180(1):99–107.

28. Keels E, Sethna N, Watterberg KL, et al. Prevention and management of procedural pain in the neonate: an update. Pediatrics 2016;137(2). https://doi.org/10.1542/peds.2015-4271.

29. Anand KJS, International Evidence-Based Group for Neonatal Pain. Consensus statement for the prevention and management of pain in the newborn. Arch Pediatr Adolesc Med 2001;155(2):173.

30. Lago P, Garetti E, Merazzi D, et al. Guidelines for procedural pain in the newborn. Acta Paediatr 2009;98(6):932–9.

31. Campbell-Yeo M, Eriksson M, Benoit B. Assessment and management of pain in preterm infants: a practice update. Children 2022;9(2):244.

32. Eriksson M, Campbell-Yeo M. Assessment of pain in newborn infants. Semin Fetal Neonatal Med 2019;24(4):101003.

33. Meesters N, Dilles T, Simons S, et al. Do pain measurement instruments detect the effect of pain-reducing interventions in neonates? a systematic review on responsiveness. J Pain 2019;20(7):760–70.

34. Franck LS, Ridout D, Howard R, et al. A comparison of pain measures in newborn infants after cardiac surgery. Pain 2011;152(8):1758–65.

35. Mörelius E, Theodorsson E, Nelson N. Stress at three-month immunization: parents' and infants' salivary cortisol response in relation to the use of pacifier and oral glucose. Eur J Pain 2009;13(2):202–8.

36. Jones L, Laudiano-Dray MP, Whitehead K, et al. The impact of parental contact upon cortical noxious-related activity in human neonates. Eur J Pain 2021;25(1): 149–59.

37. Fabrizi L, Worley A, Patten D, et al. Electrophysiological measurements and analysis of nociception in human infants. JoVE 2011;58. https://doi.org/10.3791/3118.

38. Goksan S, Hartley C, Emery F, et al. fMRI reveals neural activity overlap between adult and infant pain. Elife 2015;4. https://doi.org/10.7554/eLife.06356.

39. Bellieni CV, Bagnoli F, Sisto R, et al. Development and validation of the ABC pain scale for healthy full-term babies. Acta Paediatr 2007;94(10):1432–6.

40. Holsti L, Grunau RE. Initial validation of the behavioural indicators of infant pain (BIIP). Pain 2007;132(3):264–72.

41. Schenk K, Stoffel L, Bürgin R, et al. The influence of gestational age in the psychometric testing of the Bernese Pain Scale for Neonates. BMC Pediatr 2019; 19(1):20.

42. Schenk K, Stoffel L, Bürgin R, et al. Acute pain measured with the modified Bernese Pain Scale for Neonates is influenced by individual contextual factors. Eur J Pain 2020;24(6):1107–18.

43. Olsson E, Ahl H, Bengtsson K, et al. The use and reporting of neonatal pain scales: a systematic review of randomized trials. Pain 2021;162(2):353–60.

44. Milesi C, Cambonie G, Jacquot A, et al. Validation of a neonatal pain scale adapted to the new practices in caring for preterm newborns. Arch Dis Child Fetal Neonatal Ed 2010;95(4):F263–6.

45. Merkel SI, Voepel-Lewis T, Shayevitz JR, et al. The FLACC: a behavioural scale for scoring postoperative pain in young children. Pediatr Nurs 1997;23(3):293–7.

46. Grunau RVE, Craig KD. Pain expression in neonates: facial action and cry. Pain 1987;28(3):395–410.

47. Lawrence J, Alcock D, McGrath P, et al. The development of a tool to assess neonatal pain. Neonatal Netw 1993;12(6):59–66.

48. Pölkki T, Korhonen A, Axelin A, et al. Development and preliminary validation of the neonatal infant acute pain assessment scale (NIAPAS). Int J Nurs Stud 2014; 51(12):1585–94.

49. Stevens BJ, Gibbins S, Yamada J, et al. The premature infant pain profile-revised (PIPP-R). Clin J Pain 2014;30(3):238–43.

50. Stevens B, Johnston C, Petryshen P, et al. Premature infant pain profile: development and initial validation. Clin J Pain 1996;12(1):13–22.

51. Hummel P, Puchalski M, Creech SD, et al. Clinical reliability, and validity of the N-PASS: neonatal pain, agitation, and sedation scale with prolonged pain. J Perinatol 2008;28(1):55–60.

52. Hodgkinson K, Bear M, Thorn J, et al. Measuring pain in neonates: evaluating an instrument and developing a common language. Aust J Adv Nurs 1994;12(1): 17–22.

53. Lundqvist P, Kleberg A, Edberg A, et al. Development and psychometric properties of the S Swedish ALPS - N to pain and stress assessment scale for newborn infants. Acta Paediatr 2014;103(8):833–9.

54. van Dijk M, Roofthooft DWE, Anand KJS, et al. Taking up the challenge of measuring prolonged pain in (premature) neonates. Clin J Pain 2009;25(7): 607–16.

55. Debillon T, Zupan V, Ravault N, et al. Development and initial validation of the EDIN scale, a new tool for assessing prolonged pain in preterm infants. Arch Dis Child Fetal Neonatal Ed 2001;85(1):36F–41F.

56. Ramelet AS, Rees N, Mcdonald S, et al. Development and preliminary psychometric testing of the multidimensional assessment of pain scale: MAPS. Pediatric Anesthesia 2007;17(4):333–40.

57. Hall RW, Anand KJS. Pain management in newborns. Clin Perinatol 2014;41(4): 895–924.

58. Witt N, Coynor S, Edwards C, et al. A guide to pain assessment and management in the neonate. Curr Emerg Hosp Med Rep 2016;4:1–10.

59. Marín Gabriel MÁ, del Rey Hurtado de Mendoza B, Jiménez Figueroa L, et al. Analgesia with breastfeeding in addition to skin-to-skin contact during heel prick. Arch Dis Child Fetal Neonatal Ed 2013;98(6):F499–503.

60. Roué JM. Assessment of neonatal pain. Uptodate. Published online 2023.

61. Shen Q, Huang Z, Leng H, et al. Efficacy and safety of non-pharmacological interventions for neonatal pain: an overview of systematic reviews. BMJ Open 2022;12(9):e062296.

62. Maciel HIA, Costa MF, Costa ACL, et al. Pharmacological and nonpharmacological measures of pain management and treatment among neonates. Rev Bras Ter Intensiva 2019;31(1):21–6.

63. Benoit B, Martin-Misener R, Latimer M, et al. Breast-feeding analgesia in infants. J Perinat Neonatal Nurs 2017;31(2):145–59.

64. Shah PS, Herbozo C, Aliwalas LL, et al. Breastfeeding or breast milk for procedural pain in neonates. Cochrane Database Syst Rev 2012;2012(12). https://doi.org/10.1002/14651858.CD004950.pub3.

65. Shah V, Taddio A, McMurtry CM, et al. Pharmacological and combined interventions to reduce vaccine injection pain in children and adults. Clin J Pain 2015;31(Supplement 10):S38–63.

66. Weissman A, Aranovitch M, Blazer S, et al. Heel-lancing in newborns: behavioural and spectral analysis assessment of pain control methods. Pediatrics 2009;124(5):e921–6.

67. Johnston C, Campbell-Yeo M, Disher T, et al. Skin-to-skin care for procedural pain in neonates. Cochrane Database Syst Rev 2017;2017(2). https://doi.org/10.1002/14651858.CD008435.pub3.

68. Gao H, Xu G, Gao H, et al. Effect of repeated kangaroo mother care on repeated procedural pain in preterm infants: a randomized controlled trial. Int J Nurs Stud 2015;52(7):1157–65.

69. Shukla VV, Chaudhari AJ, Nimbalkar SM, et al. Skin-to-skin care by mother vs. father for preterm neonatal pain: a randomized control trial (ENVIRON Trial). Int J Pediatr 2021;2021:8886887.

70. Ferreira A, Ferretti E, Curtis K, et al. Parents' views to strengthen partnerships in newborn intensive care. Front Pediatr 2021;9. https://doi.org/10.3389/fped.2021.721835.

71. Orovou E, Tzitiridou-Chatzopoulou M, Dagla M, et al. Correlation between pacifier use in preterm neonates and breastfeeding in infancy: a systematic review. Children 2022;9(10). https://doi.org/10.3390/children9101585.

72. Pillai Riddell RR, Bucsea O, Shiff I, et al. Non-pharmacological management of infant and young child procedural pain. Cochrane Database Syst Rev 2023;2023(6). https://doi.org/10.1002/14651858.CD006275.pub4.

73. Carbajal R, Rousset A, Danan C, et al. Epidemiology and treatment of painful procedures in neonates in intensive care units. JAMA 2008;300(1):60.

74. Erkut Z, Yildiz S. The effect of swaddling on pain, vital signs, and crying duration during heel lance in newborns. Pain Manag Nurs 2017;18(5):328–36.

75. Liaw JJ, Yang L, Katherine Wang KW, et al. Non-nutritive sucking and facilitated tucking relieve preterm infant pain during heel-stick procedures: a prospective, randomised controlled crossover trial. Int J Nurs Stud 2012;49(3):300–9.

76. Gomes Neto M, da Silva Lopes IA, Araujo ACCLM, et al. The effect of facilitated tucking position during painful procedure in pain management of preterm infants in neonatal intensive care unit: a systematic review and meta-analysis. Eur J Pediatr 2020;179(5):699–709.

77. Ho LP, Ho SS, Leung DY, et al. A feasibility and efficacy randomised controlled trial of swaddling for controlling procedural pain in preterm infants. J Clin Nurs 2016;25(3–4):472–82.

78. Stevens B, Yamada J, Ohlsson A, et al. Sucrose for analgesia in newborn infants undergoing painful procedures. Cochrane Database Syst Rev 2016;2017(2). https://doi.org/10.1002/14651858.CD001069.pub5.

79. Collados-Gómez L, Ferrera-Camacho P, Fernandez-Serrano E, et al. Randomised crossover trial showed that using breast milk or sucrose provided the same analgesic effect in preterm infants of at least 28 weeks. Acta Paediatr 2018;107(3):436–41.

80. Kumar P, Sharma R, Rathour S, et al. Effectiveness of various nonpharmacological analgesic methods in newborns. Clin Exp Pediatr 2020;63(1):25–9.

81. Mangat AK, Oei JL, Chen K, et al. A review of non-pharmacological treatments for pain management in newborn infants. Children 2018;5(10). https://doi.org/10.3390/children5100130.

82. Harrison D, Larocque C, Bueno M, et al. Sweet solutions to reduce procedural pain in neonates: a meta-analysis. Pediatrics 2017;139(1). https://doi.org/10.1542/peds.2016-0955.

83. Bellieni CV, Cordelli DM, Marchi S, et al. Sensorial saturation for neonatal analgesia. Clin J Pain 2007;23(3):219–21.

84. Stevens B, Yamada J, Campbell-Yeo M, et al. The minimally effective dose of sucrose for procedural pain relief in neonates: a randomized controlled trial. BMC Pediatr 2018;18(1):85.

85. Balice-Bourgois C, Zumstein-Shaha M, Vanoni F, et al. A systematic review of clinical practice guidelines for acute procedural pain on neonates. Clin J Pain 2020;36(5):390–8.

86. Kinoshita M, Olsson E, Borys F, et al. Opioids for procedural pain in neonates. Cochrane Database Syst Rev 2023;2023(4). https://doi.org/10.1002/14651858.CD015056.pub2.

87. Bellù R, Romantsik O, Nava C, et al. Opioids for newborn infants receiving mechanical ventilation. Cochrane Database Syst Rev 2021;2021(3). https://doi.org/10.1002/14651858.CD013732.pub2.

88. Stróżyk A, Paraskevas T, Romantsik O, et al. Pharmacological pain and sedation interventions for the prevention of intraventricular hemorrhage in preterm infants on assisted ventilation - an overview of systematic reviews. Cochrane Database Syst Rev 2023;2023(8). https://doi.org/10.1002/14651858.CD012706.pub2.

89. Barrington K, Batton D, Finley G, et al. Canadian paediatric society fetus and newborn committee. prevention and management of pain in the neonate: an update. Pediatrics 2006;118(5):2231–41.

90. Ohlsson A, Shah PS. Paracetamol (acetaminophen) for prevention or treatment of pain in newborns. Cochrane Database Syst Rev 2016;10(10):CD011219.

91. Aldrink JH, Ma M, Wang W, et al. Safety of ketorolac in surgical neonates and infants 0 to 3 months old. J Pediatr Surg 2011;46(6):1081–5.

92. Ziesenitz VC, Welzel T, van Dyk M, et al. Efficacy and safety of NSAIDs in infants: a comprehensive review of the literature of the past 20 years. Pediatr Drugs 2022;24(6):603–55.

93. Carter BS, Brunkhorst J. Neonatal pain management. Semin Perinatol 2017;41(2):111–6.

94. Persad E, Pizarro AB, Bruschettini M. Non-opioid analgesics for procedural pain in neonates. Cochrane Database Syst Rev 2023;2023(4). https://doi.org/10.1002/14651858.CD015179.pub2.

95. Mantecón-Fernández L, Lareu-Vidal S, González-López C, et al. An alternative to pain treatment in neonatology. Children 2023;10(3):454.

96. Ojha S, Abramson J, Dorling J. Sedation and analgesia from prolonged pain and stress during mechanical ventilation in preterm infants: is dexmedetomidine an alternative to current practice? BMJ Paediatr Open 2022;6(1):e001460.

97. Foster JP, Taylor C, Spence K. Topical anaesthesia for needle-related pain in newborn infants. Cochrane Database Syst Rev 2017;2017(2). https://doi.org/10.1002/14651858.CD010331.pub2.

98. Shavit I, Peri-Front Y, Rosen-Walther A, et al. A randomized trial to evaluate the effect of two topical anesthetics on pain response during frenotomy in young infants. Pain Med 2017;18(2):356–62.

99. Labban M, Menhem Z, Bandali T, et al. Pain control in neonatal male circumcision: a best evidence review. J Pediatr Urol 2021;17(1):3–8.

100. Dempsey E, McCreery K. Local anaesthetic eye drops for prevention of pain in preterm infants undergoing screening for retinopathy of prematurity. Cochrane Database Syst Rev 2011. https://doi.org/10.1002/14651858.CD007645.pub2. Published online September 7.

101. Disher T, Cameron C, Mitra S, et al. Pain-relieving interventions for retinopathy of prematurity: a meta-analysis. Pediatrics 2018;142(1). https://doi.org/10.1542/peds.2018-0401.

102. Kinoshita M, Stempel KS, Borges do Nascimento IJ, et al. Systemic opioids versus other analgesics and sedatives for postoperative pain in neonates. Cochrane Database Syst Rev 2023;2023(3). https://doi.org/10.1002/14651858.CD014876.pub2.

103. Donato J, Rao K, Lewis T. Pharmacology of common analgesic and sedative drugs used in the neonatal intensive care unit. Clin Perinatol 2019;46(4):673–92.

104. Ng E, Taddio A, Ohlsson A. Intravenous midazolam infusion for sedation of infants in the neonatal intensive care unit. Cochrane Database Syst Rev 2017. https://doi.org/10.1002/14651858.CD002052.pub3.

105. American Association on Intellectual and Developmental Disabilities. Defining criteria for intellectual disability. Published online 2022.

106. Barney CC, Andersen RD, Defrin R, et al. Challenges in pain assessment and management among individuals with intellectual and developmental disabilities. Pain Rep 2020;5(4):e821.

107. Abanto J, Ciamponi AL, Francischini E, et al. Medical problems and oral care of patients with Down syndrome: a literature review. Spec Care Dentist 2011;31(6):197–203.

108. Henderson A, Lynch SA, Wilkinson S, et al. Adults with Down's syndrome: the prevalence of complications and health care in the community. Br J Gen Pract 2007;57(534):50–5.

109. Turk V, Khattran S, Kerry S, et al. Reporting of health problems and pain by adults with an intellectual disability and by their carers. J Appl Res Intellect Disabil 2012;25(2):155–65.

110. Doody O E, Bailey M. Pain and pain assessment in people with intellectual disability: issues and challenges in practice. Br J Learn Disabil 2017;45(3):157–65.

111. Daruich A, Bremond-Gignac D, Behar-Cohen F, et al. Rétinopathie du prématuré : de la prévention au traitement. M-S (Med Sci) 2020;36(10):900–7.

112. Jefferies AL, Canadian Paediatric Society, Fetus and Newborn Committee. Retinopathy of prematurity: an update on screening and management. Paediatr Child Health 2016;21(2):101–4.

113. Mitchell AJ, Green A, Jeffs DA, et al. Physiologic effects of retinopathy of prematurity screening examinations. Adv Neonatal Care 2011;11(4):291–7.

114. Gal P, Kissling GE, Young WO, et al. Efficacy of sucrose to reduce pain in premature infants during eye examinations for retinopathy of prematurity. Ann Pharmacother 2005;39(6):1029–33.

115. Sindhur M, Balasubramanian H, Srinivasan L, et al. Intranasal fentanyl for pain management during screening for retinopathy of prematurity in preterm infants: a randomized controlled trial. J Perinatol 2020;40(6):881–7.

116. Sutter MB, Leeman L, Hsi A. Neonatal opioid withdrawal syndrome. Obstet Gynecol Clin North Am 2014;41(2):317–34.

117. Stevens B, Riahi S, Cardoso R, et al. The influence of context on pain practices in the nicu: perceptions of health care professionals. Qual Health Res 2011; 21(6):757–70.

118. Hamers J, Zimmermann L, van Lingen RA, et al. Neonatal procedural pain exposure and pain management in ventilated preterm infants during the first 14 days of life. Swiss Med Wkly 2009. https://doi.org/10.4414/smw.2009.12545.

119. Bäcke P, Bruschettini M, Blomqvist YT, et al. Interventions for the management of pain and sedation in newborns undergoing therapeutic hypothermia for hypoxic-ischemic encephalopathy: a systematic review. Paediatr Drugs 2023; 25(1):27–41.

120. Bäcke P, Bruschettini M, Sibrecht G, et al. Pharmacological interventions for pain and sedation management in newborn infants undergoing therapeutic hypothermia. Cochrane Database Syst Rev 2022;2022(11). https://doi.org/10.1002/14651858.CD015023.pub2.

What's New on the Street?
An Update on New Opioids, Psychoactive Drugs, and Synthetic Marijuana

Pamela A. Harris-Haman, DNP, APRN, NNP-BC

KEYWORDS

- Synthetic marijuana • Novel psychoactive agents • Neonatal withdrawal
- Novel opioids • Pregnancy

KEY POINTS

- Knowledge of the effects of synthetic cannabis on maternal/fetal health is limited.
- Knowledge of the effects of novel psychoactive substances on maternal/fetal health is limited.
- Novel substances are consantly emerging and present challanges for health-care providers.

INTRODUCTION

Substance abuse is a widespread problem in the United States and worldwide. The use within the pregnant population is thought to reflect a pattern similar to the general population, with estimates of 10% to 15% of pregnant women experiencing substance abuse.[1] Illicit substance use during pregnancy has increased substantially during the past decade in the United States. In 2018, an estimated 8.5% of pregnant women aged 15 to 44 years used illicit substances in the past month, reflecting a 70% increase from 2010 levels. Substance use during pregnancy is of public health concern due to potential adverse maternal and newborn health outcomes. Observational studies suggest that in utero, exposure to substances is associated with higher rates of perinatal mortality, birth defects, low birth weight, low gestational age, and neonatal drug withdrawal.[2]

During the past decade, novel or atypical substances have emerged and become increasingly popular. Recognition and treatment of new substances of abuse present many challenges for health-care providers due to a lack of quantitative reporting and surveillance. These drugs are virtually nondetectable with routine blood and urine analysis because they contain novel chemical substances.[3,4] Street manufacturers are able to manufacture and develop new synthetic isolates of older drugs.[3] These

University of Texas Medical Branch, 500 Seawall Boulevard, Unit 704, Galveston, TX 77550, USA
E-mail address: PAMHARRI@UTMB.EDU

Crit Care Nurs Clin N Am 36 (2024) 211–221
https://doi.org/10.1016/j.cnc.2023.12.002
0899-5885/24/© 2023 Elsevier Inc. All rights reserved.

novel drugs are not necessarily new inventions but have recently been made available. Newer drugs can include a failed pharmaceutical or an old patent that has been redis-covered and marketed for its potential use as a recreational substance. Conversely, the term novel can also express something newly created or a compound that has come back into fashion after a period of absence from the recreational drug scene. These substances are often more affordable, more easily acquired, and lack the stigma associated with other substances of abuse.[3,5]

NOVEL PSYCHOACTIVE SUBSTANCES

Novel psychoactive substances (NPSs) represent a heterogenous family of substances, including synthetic cannabimimetics, synthetic cathinones, phenethylamines, ketamine, piperazine, tryptamines, psychoactive plants and herbs, prescribed medications, novel stimulants, and synthetic opioids.[6–8]

NPSs mimic the effects of recreational drugs with psychoactive effects.[6] NPSs are more easily available at lower processing costs; they may be a known psychoactive substance being used in a novel way, are usually legalized, and cannot be detected in mandatory drug screens.[3,6,9] They are often commercialized as "legal highs" or "smart drugs" and are advertised as "safer" or "legal" alternatives to illicit or controlled drugs.[3,9] NPSs are often not routinely part of the health history and remain undis-closed or undetected during pregnancy.[10]

Synthetic Cannabimimetic

Synthetic cannabimimetics are CB-1 and CB-2 receptor agonists that display a higher affinity, efficacy, and potency than Δ 9-tetrahydrocannabinol (THC).[11] Synthetic can-nabimimetics are unrelated to THC structurally but stimulate the same receptors. Syn-thetic cannabinoids are mind-altering chemicals or mixtures of chemicals structurally related to Δ 9-THC that are sprayed on dried, shredded plant material and sold. They are much more powerful than cannabis or Δ 9-THC, sometimes more than 100 times stronger with potent psychoactivity and likely with a myriad of other known and un-known adverse health effects on the human body.[12]

Typically sold as herbal smoking mixtures or liquid incense in metal-foil packets, these products containing chemicals are mostly manufactured in China.[3,8,11,12] Once shipped, the powder is dissolved in a solvent, such as acetone, ethanol, embalming fluid,[11] or methanol, and sprayed onto the herbs. It is then left to dry, leav-ing behind a "natural" product. This is then packaged for sale. Consumers are given the impression they are smoking a "natural herbal" product.[3,8,11,12]

Although low-level dosages of synthetic cannabinoids produce similar psychoactive effects to those of cannabis and THC, with higher dosages, auditory and visual halluci-nations, anxiety, and intense feelings of paranoia often occur. Other psychiatric and neurologic effects include agitation, mood swings, and suicidal ideation. Suicide at-tempts, panic attacks, disorganization, and persistent psychotic disorders have been described. The acute intoxication toxic effects seem to be similar to those experienced with sympathomimetic stimulant drug use. Typical medical side effects include vomiting and nausea, hypertension, hyperglycemia, mydriasis, seizures, encephalopathy, coma, and stroke. Ultimately, deaths have been associated with the use of synthetic cannabi-noids, either on their own or in combination with other substances.[5]

Kratom

Kratom has been used in Thailand for centuries. Newer herbal products such as Kra-tom are gaining popularity and are being widely used in the United States. Touted as a natural herbal product, Kratom is misconceived as a safe alternative for opioids by its users.[3] Its biologically active alkaloids, mitragyna (MG), and 7-hydroxy mitragynine bind and stimulate the μ receptors. Kratom is a member of the *Mitragyna speciosa* tree and is a member of the same family as the coffee plant.[3] Its predominant active component, MG is a known μ opioid agonist and is a Food and Drug Administration drug of concern. Kratom is not classified and is sold as compressed tablets, liquid for oral administration, loose leaves for smoking and steeping, and whole leaves for chewing. Kratom can be found in US vape shops and smoke shops, is frequently referred to as gas station heroin, and is sold as a dietary supplement. Products in the United States are not the same as the traditionally used "fresh leaves."[3] Kratom is thought by some to have therapeutic potential; however, there is no standardized protocol for manufacturing the product. Kratom is known to increase energy, reduce anxiety, decrease pain, and reduce opioid withdrawal. Lower doses produce mild stimulation, and higher doses are associated with sedation. Associated symptoms are hyperpigmentation of skin on the cheeks, constipation, weight loss, insomnia, xerostomia, limited sexual desire, agitation, irritability, diarrhea, hyperventilation, and tachypnea.[13,14] Kratom may be reversed by naloxone; however, it is not detectable in standard drug screens[3] (**Table 1**).

Synthetic Cathinones

Synthetic cathinones and methcathinones are NPSs marketed under the generic title of bath salts. Psychoactive bath salts may contain one drug or a mixture of several psychoactive drugs.[1] The most popular bath salt constituents include mephedrone, methyl-one, and 3,4-methylenedioxypyrovalerone. During the past few years, attention has been drawn to mephedrone.[1] Cathinones act at the dopamine (DA), serotonin (5-HT), and norepinephrine (NA) synapses and produce stimulant-like effects similar to methamphetamines and cocaine. Cathinones exert an inhibitory action on monoamine reuptake, increasing the quantity of DA, NA, and 5-HT, molecules that present with high

Table 1
Synthetic cannabinoids[3,5,7,9]

Substance	Behavioral/ Psychological Associations	Intoxication/Acute Toxic Affects	Long Term Effects
Spice, K2, Krypton, Fake weed	Hallucinations Anxiety Paranoia Agitation mood swings Suicidal ideation Panic attacks	Vomiting/nausea, hypertension, tachycardia, tachypnea, dyspnea, encephalopathy, coma, stroke, seizures, nystagmus, acute kidney injury (without prior history) abdominal or flank pain, elevated creatinine, and blood urea nitrogen (BUN), and predisposition to end-stage renal disease in later life	Dependence, tolerance, withdrawal, profuse sweating, tachycardia, tremors, headache, diarrhea, feeling depressed, and nightmares
Kava, *Piper methysticum*	Depressant Used for stress relief, antianxiolytic		Shrub or root Found in vape oil Considered a dietary supplement and as such is not regulated

5-HT-DA ratios and may be considered analogous to entactogenic substances such as methylenedioxymethamphetamine (MDMA), more commonly known as ecstasy.[4,14]

MDPV is 10 times more potent than cocaine and produces a cocaine-like blockage of transporters for DA and NA.[15] Intake of these substances is typically associated with an imbalance of a range of neurotransmitter pathways/receptors and, therefore, are associated with a risk of psychopathological disturbances.[5] Cathinone-induced acute intoxication may include symptoms of serotonin syndrome, hyperthermia, psychotic disorders, catatonia, dehydration, hypertension, tachycardia, kidney and liver impairment, electrolyte imbalance, and cerebral edema. Suicides by hanging and deaths from firearm injuries have been reported, as well as deaths from toxicity.

Novel stimulants and novel psychedelic compounds include phenethylamines, piperazines, cathinones, and amphetamines. Phenethylamines are NPSs that are 5-HT receptor agonists and inhibit monoamine reuptake. Piperazines are stimulants that promote the release of DA and noradrenaline and inhibit monoamine reuptake.[11]

All these present with varying levels of stimulant and hallucinogenic effects. With mephedrone, low mood, loss of appetite, difficulty sleeping, levels of paranoia, ideation, cognitive impairment changes, perception, agitation, hallucination, delusions, amnesia, confusion, violence, and suicidal thoughts have been reported. Users reported euphoria, improved psychomotor speed, alertness, and talkativeness.

Long-term use can lead to a dependence tolerance phenomenon, a withdrawal syndrome characterized by profuse, sweating, tachycardia, tremor, diarrhea, headache, drug craving, depression, insomnia, nightmares, and anxiety have been described.

Over-the-Counter Medications

Over-the-counter (OTC) drugs include ephedra, pseudoephedrine, and dextromethorphan. The psychotropic effects and addictive potential are associated with the intake of larger doses typically administered through snorting. Psychotropic effects include euphoria or stupor, hyperexcitability, depersonalization, dyskinesia, delayed response times, disordered speech, visual and auditory hallucinations, and may produce a dissociative state. Acute intoxication has been linked to serotonin syndrome, especially if used together with other serotonergic agents. Recently, the antidiarrheal compound, loperamide, has been reported for its euphoric effects. Therapeutic loperamide doses of 2 to 16 mg per day are considered safe due to both rapid metabolism and poor blood–brain barrier penetration. However, when self-administered at higher doses of more than 50 mg, its μ opioid receptor agonist activities explain why loperamide, or "Lope," as it is referred to on the street, has been anecdotally described as better than oxycodone.[5] Loperamide has been linked to central nervous system depression and fatal cardiotoxicity. Standard toxicity tests can identify just a few misused molecules, and only expensive, lengthy tests carried out in specialized settings are able to identify the vast range of NPSs available.

Khat/Qat

Khat is a stimulant grown in East Africa and the Arab peninsula and has been chewed for thousands of years. Known for its euphoric and stimulant-like properties (much like coffee), it is thought by many that it is grown to have health benefits.[3] Cathinones and cathines are naturally occurring drugs extracted from the Khat plant. Beginning around 2007, there was an explosion in the availability of synthetic analogs of cathinone, reportedly developed in China and India, with these drugs becoming available in large quantities in Europe. This new trend of designer drugs quickly spread to the United States.[1] Khat is not illegal but cathinone (a drug that is in the leaves) is a Schedule 1 drug, making it regulated in the United States[3] (**Table 2**).

Table 2
Synthetic cathiones[3,5,7,9,14]

Substance	Behavioral/Psychoactive Associations	Toxic Affects	Long-Term Effects
Novel stimulants/ psychedelics Cathinones, Khat, bath salts	Low mood, paranoia, cognitive impairment, changes in perception, agitation, aggression, hallucinations, delusions, amnesia, catatonia, excited delirium, confusion, violence, suicidal ideation, increased incidence of suicides by hanging and deaths by firearms	Serotonin syndrome, hyperthermia, dehydration, tachycardia, hypertension, kidney and liver impairment, electrolyte imbalance, metabolic toxicity, cerebral edema, rhabdomyolysis, stroke, respiratory illness, and myocardial infarction	Insomnia, depression, anxiety, psychosis, dependence, largely unknown
Phenethylamines	Hallucinations and anxiety	Loss of appetite, tachycardia, hypertension, nausea, headache, dizziness, skin irritation, hyperthermia, convulsions, respiratory deficits, liver/kidney failure, and death	
Piperazines	Hallucinations	Hyperthermia, kidney failure, seizures, hyponatremia, serotonin syndrome, renal failure, and death	
Tryptamines	Visual hallucinations, alterations in sensory perceptions, distortion of body image, agitation, depersonalization, and marked mood liability	Tachycardia, serotonin syndrome, and hyperpyrexia	

NOVEL OPIOIDS

Novel synthetic opioids (NSOs) have emerged in recent years as part of the worldwide opioid crisis. NSOs are a large group of narcotic analgesic drugs having structural similarities but much greater potency of action and receptor affinity with respect to morphine. They are produced at lower costs, stronger or longer lasting highs and are capable of being synthesized very efficiently.[4] This group includes compounds that were originally synthesized by pharmaceutical companies but never commercialized and then diverted into the illegal market. These molecules may be used alone as adulterants to heroin or as constituents of other illicit products or counterfeit medications.

NSO toxicity includes disorientation, slurred speech, confusion, dizziness, nausea, meiosis, sedation, euphoria, feeling of relaxation, mood lift, dysphoric and disassociating effects, slowed breathing, and respiratory depression due to their high potency. Their continued use or abuse may induce tolerance, with the risk of overdose and death being elevated. Physical dependence and addiction may rapidly develop, and withdrawal symptoms occur if their use is rapidly reduced or suddenly stopped.[3,5,8] Their detection can be difficult as they often have novel chemical structures.[4]

Ketamine

Ketamine can induce feelings of relaxation, disassociation, depersonalization, and psychotic experiences, with hallucinations lasting even longer than the anesthetic effects. Ketamine intoxication may include cardiovascular and respiratory symptoms due to its anesthetic effects. The risks of these associative effects may include trauma, drowning, death from hypothermia, and traffic accidents. The "keyhole," which may result from the ingestion of large doses of ketamine, is a typical out-of-body near-death experience, with the user becoming trapped in a state of detachment from his or her physical presence. In the long term, it can lead to both urologic bladder and intestinal cramping syndromes.[5]

Carfentanyl

Carfentanyl has a high potency that is 10,000 times more potent than morphine. It has a rapid onset of action and a long half-life. Initially, it circulated in the mid-1980s as a general anesthetic for large animals, such as elephants.[4] The ease of synthesis of carfentanyl makes it a low-cost additive and is often mixed with other drugs to improve their potency; the user may be unaware of the addition.[3] Opioids xylazine and carfentanyl are frequently laced with or disguised as heroin.[8]

Krokidile

Krokidile or desomorphine is a morphine-like analog with high potency and is fast acting and of short duration.[3] Krokidile produces opioid-like effects and may cause disorientation, confusion, respiratory depression, coma, and death. Injection has been shown to produce ulcers at the injection sites, rapid systemic infections, and gangrene. Home chemists often start with codeine and use organic solvents such as gasoline, paint thinner, iodine, or hydrochloric acid to make the substance. Other components may also be used because it is a home-based manufactured product.[3] If the drug is mixed with other drugs, the effects may be worse.[3]

Gabapentinoids

Gabapentinoids bind to the calcium channel, reducing the release of excitatory molecules. They are rapidly absorbed, have a faster onset of action, and attain maximum plasma concentrations and bioavailability.[6] At therapeutic doses, they are thought to possess gamma memetic properties, which may be behind the liking or euphoric, relaxing high but causing only limited rewarding or wanting properties. A range of experiences may be associated with gabapentinoids, including euphoria, improved social ability, opiate-like sedation, disassociation, and psychedelic effects. Gabapentinoids may be ingested to cope with opiate or opioid withdrawal symptoms and have a high abuse potential. Unconventional routes of administration have been reported, such as bugging, smoking, and parachuting, which is emptying the contents of a capsule into a pouch[6] **(Table 3)**.

Table 3
Novel opioids[5,8,11,13,14,16]

Substance	Psychoactive Affects	Toxic Affects	Long-Term Effects	Other
Desomorphine, krokodil, and carfentanyl	Sedation Disorientation Euphoria Dissociating effect Confusion, dizziness	Nausea, miosis Slowed breathing Drowsiness, slurred speech, nausea, respiratory depression to coma, powder	Tolerance withdrawal symptoms (Muscle and bone pain, insomnia, diarrhea, vomiting, and cold flashes)	Alveolar hemorrhage after insufflating fentanyl
Ketamine-like dissociative-Special K	Relaxation, disassociation, depersonalization, psychotic experiences	Cardiovascular and respiratory effects related to its anesthetic and dissociative effects Trauma, drowning, hypothermia, and traffic accidents	K-bladder K-cramps	
Gabapentinoids	Euphoria, anxiety, compulsions, improved sociability Opiate-like sedation, psychedelic effects, and hallucinations	Insomnia, irritability, headache, and nausea	Used to cope with opioid withdrawal effects	Unconventional routes of administration (rectal plugging, smoking, and parachuting)

MATERNAL/FETAL EFFECTS

Exogenous cannabinoids such as Δ 9-THC have been shown to cross the fetal–placental barrier in humans. Cannabinoids' effect on the growth and development of the fetus, as well as learning, memory, neuronal, behavioral, and endocrine aspects of the infant's development, have been studied and reviewed. Perinatal intrauterine exposure may profoundly alter the fetal immune system, suggesting that cannabis exposure during pregnancy may cause significant and long-lasting effects on immune function.[12]

The anti-inflammatory activity of cannabinoids can have a significant impact during pregnancy. Nonsteroidal anti-inflammatory drugs (NSAIDs) used during pregnancy have been linked to miscarriages and adverse outcomes. Exposure to NSAIDs during the third trimester can affect fetal development and cause fetal ductal constriction.[12] Synthetic cannabinoids have been shown to potentially reduce placental blood flow, and they may create effects similar to preeclampsia and eclampsia. High protein levels have been noted in pregnant women who use synthetic cannabinoids along with high blood pressure medication. Identified effects in children born to women who have used synthetic cannabinoids include learning disabilities, cortical developmental deficits, attention deficit hyperactivity disorder (ADHD), aggression, anxiety, and depression that are noted to last into the teenage years.[12,16] It has also been postulated that synthetic cannabinoids may produce epigenetic changes in maternal DNA and microRNA influencing neuronal, immune systems, and inflammatory mediators. These changes may then be transferred to her offspring leading to a direct and heritable impact on neuronal and immune systems. The subsequent impact on the offspring could include behavioral and cognitive impairments, immune dysfunction, and impaired immune responses to infections and cancer.[12]

Kratom uses in pregnancy and its effects on the developing fetus and newborn are largely unknown.[16] No published studies exist regarding the safety and efficacy of kratom for maternal use or its effect on the fetus during pregnancy.[17] Kratom may cause withdrawal symptoms in the infant, per a report by Davidson and colleagues. Deaths have been reported, although there was an association with the mixing of another substance with kratom.[3] Women of childbearing age are using kratom and becoming pregnant without knowing or being advised of the consequences of continued use during pregnancy. The publicized claims refer to kratom as being nonaddictive or a safe alternative to opioids that do not present a risk to mothers. Kratom is "legal" and therefore not reported, leading to public misinterpretation of the safety of prenatal exposure.[10]

There is virtually no information on NPSs use in pregnancy; only a few small case studies exist.[15] Cathinones are known to cause narrowing of blood vessels, resulting in decreased blood flow. A possible link has been associated with the use of cathinones and gastroschisis.[11] Pregnancy taxes the cardiovascular system, likely affecting blood pressure and uterine blood flow. Increased cardiovascular stress resulting from NPSs exposure, resulting in tachycardia and hypertension, is difficult to distinguish from preeclampsia. Differentiating between eclampsia and drug-induced seizures is often difficult.[1,15] Synthetic cathinones have also been associated with hyperthermia in the user. Hyperthermia in pregnancy is defined as a temperature greater than 101°F. Severe hyperthermia can cause fetal death and spontaneous abortion, as well as fetal anomalies. Hyperthermia with potential rhabdomyolysis, renal failure, impaired liver function, and metabolic acidosis will produce a dangerous intrauterine environment for the fetus. Blood pressure alterations may be produced by cathinone, which can include hypertension, hyperreflexia, and muscle twitching, as seen with preeclampsia.[1]

Pregnant women who use MDMA are more likely to suffer negative consequences during pregnancy, including work and social problems. Infants born to these women are more likely to have congenital anomalies and musculoskeletal malformations than the general population. Its use in pregnancy has also been associated with vasoconstrictive disorders such as gastroschisis.[15]

Venlafaxine (Effexor, Morrisville, NC) is an antidepressant medication that is a pregnancy C-category drug. Its use is not advised in pregnancy; however, there have been very few studies on pregnant women. Venlafaxine is rarely available in pure form, often being mixed with other drugs. These added drugs may be harmful to the mother or infant.[11] Olanzapine (Zyprexa, Cambridge, MA), an atypical antipsychotic drug, is a category C drug and has been noted to cause hyperglycemia in pregnant women. The concern is how this will prevent the fetus from seeing higher-than-normal glucose levels. Normal physiology dictates that the fetus will produce an increased insulin load in response to maternal hyperglycemia, thus leading to an infant at risk for complications of hyperinsulinemia. The potential for withdrawal symptoms has also been noted in the infants of women who used olanzapine. There are no other noted risks associated with pregnancy.[9] Loperamide is a pregnancy C-category drug and is harmless when taken as advised. Taken in higher doses, it is known to cause cardiotoxicity and arrhythmias. Characteristics of the arrhythmias have included widened QRS complex and QT interval prolongation. The effects on the fetus are unknown. However, concern for maternal cardiac function and placental blood flow should be considered.[11]

NPSs affect the balance of chemicals in the brain. The ability to breastfeed may also be affected because NPSs may affect milk supply. NPSs do transfer into breast milk and can cause loss of appetite in the mother. They may cause a decrease in the ability of the mother to care for her infant.[11] The many and varied NPSs on the market make it difficult to obtain data. There is no available information on the prevalence of cathinones "bath salt" use among pregnant women.[15] This may be due to underreporting or lack of knowledge on the part of the providers. Many of the new compounds are not detectable in the routine screenings.[11,15]

Khat chewing during pregnancy is associated with maternal anemia, stillbirths, prematurity, and low birth weights.[2] In the areas where Khat is grown, there is a high consumption rate (40% of pregnant women) because it is thought to have many beneficial effects such as headache relief and assisting with birth and delivery. However, Khat is also known in these areas to increase postimplantation losses, be teratogenic, cause intrauterine growth restriction (IUGR), diminish APGAR scores, decrease maternal myometrial blood flow, and increase the risk of a dysmature infant.[1,3,13] In lactating women who chew, Khat or pseudoephedrine has been found in their breast milk. If other chemicals have been added in the manufacturing, these may have adverse effects on mother and baby depending on the chemical. These substances may include organic solvents and heavy metals.[5]

Ketamine use is contraindicated in pregnancy before term due to the oxytocic activity. It is also contraindicated in patients with eclampsia or preeclampsia and may lead to premature birth and developmental delay. No studies have been done to see if it passes in human milk.[1] Gabapentinoids are a category C drug and are not advised for use in pregnancy. They are secreted in human milk and may affect milk production; however, the effects on newborns are unknown.[1] The potency and efficacy of synthetic opioids increase overdose potential and have raised fatalities. The recommended dose of naloxone does not seem to be effective enough at reviving the effects of synthetic opioids.[18]

SUMMARY

Given the unknown and potentially untoward effect these substances may have on the mother and infant, caution should be raised as to how this may affect the fetus and the potential effects following birth. Health-care providers need to be familiar with the potential effects of these substances on the mother, fetus, and infant when born. Many of these substances are being used increasingly as self-treatment or as "opioid" alternatives in pregnant women.[9] These substances are often not detectable on routine toxicology screens, and many are sold as OTC or nutritional supplements, leading to incorrect information regarding the effects of the substances on the mother and infant. Any substance exposure for the growing fetus may have effects, some that are known and some that are not. However, the net effects on newborn health are uncertain and will depend on the intensity of use and toxicities between substituted substances.[2] Occurrence of toxicity and untoward fetal effects from designer drug use must be kept high on the watch list for all who practice in maternal–fetal, newborn, and emergency departments.[1]

CLINICS CARE POINTS

- Many novel substances are not detectable in routine meconium, blood, and urine tests.
- Recognition of new drugs of abuse presents a challenge to providers.
- Many of the toxic effects of the novel substances can mimic pregnancy-associated problems such as preeclampsia and eclampsia.
- Many substances are marked as safe for use or herbal/nutritional supplements.
- Many providers are not aware of the potential complications of these substances.

DISCLOSURE

The author has nothing to disclose.

REFERENCES

1. Gray B, Holland C. Implications of psychoactive" Bath Salts" use during pregnancy. Nursing For Women's Health 2014;18(3):222–30.
2. Meinhofer A, Witman A, Maclean JC, et al. Prenatal substance use policies and newborn health. Health Econ 2022;31. https://doi.org/10.1002/hec.4518.
3. Rech M, Donahey E, Cappiello Dziedzic J, et al. New drugs of abuse. Pharmacotherapy 2015;35:2.
4. Edinoff A, Garza D, Vining S, et al. New synthetic opioids: clinical considerations and dangers. Pain Ther 2023;12:399–421.
5. Schifano F, Napoletano F, Chiappini S, et al. New/emerging psychoactive substances and associated psychopathological consequences. Psychol Med 2019;51:1.
6. Schifano F, Chiappina S, Corkey J, et al. Abuse of prescription drugs in the context of novel psychoactive substances (NPS): a systemic review. Brain Sci 2018;8:4.
7. Zawilska J, Andrzejcak D. Next generation of novel psychoactive substances on the horizon-a complex problem to face. Journal of Drug and Alcohol Dependence 2015;157. https://doi.org/10.1016/j.drugalcdep.2015.09.030.
8. Zawilska J. An expanding world of novel psychoactive substances: opioids. Front Psychiatr 2017;8:110. https://doi.org/10.3389/fpsyt.2017.00110.
9. Lovrecic B, Lovrecic M, Gabrovec B, et al. Non-medical use of novel synthetic opioids: a new challenge to public health. Int J Environ Res Publ Health 2017;16:177.

10. Wright ME, Ginsberg C, Parkinson A, et al. Outcomes of mothers and newborns to prenatal exposure to Kratom: a systematic review, 41, 2021. https://doi.org/10.1038/s41372-021-00952-8.
11. Rivera J, Vance E, Rushton W, et al. Novel psychoactive substances and trends of abuse. Crit Care Nurs Q 2017;40:4.
12. Dong C, Chen J, Harrington A, et al. Cannabinoid exposure during pregnancy and its impact on immune function. Cell Mol Life Sci 2019;76.
13. Caldwell C. Kratom and neonatal abstinence syndrome. Neonatal Network 2020; 39:1.48–49.
14. Schimmel J, Amioka E, Rockhill K, et al. Prevalence and description of kratom (mitragyna Speciosa) use in the United starts; a cross -sectional study. Addiction 2021;116. https://doi.org/10.1111/add.15082.
15. Smid M, Metz T, Gordon A. Stimulant Use in pregnancy: an under-recognized epidemic among pregnant women. Clin Obstet Gynecol 2019;62(1):168–84.
16. Eldridge W, Foster C, Wyble L. Neonatal abstinence syndrome due to maternal Kratom use. Pediatrics 2018;142:6.
17. Davidson L, Rawat M, Stojanovski S, et al. Natural drugs, not so natural effects: neonatal abstinence syndrome secondary to "kratom". J Neonatal Perinat Med 2018;12. https://doi.org/10.3233/NPM-1863.
18. Armenian P, Vo K, Barr-Walker J, et al. Fentanyl, fentanyl analogs and novel synthetic opioids: a comprehensive review. Neuropharmacology 2018;134(PtA): 121–32.

Transitioning Care Approach for Neonatal Opioid Withdrawal Syndrome and Neonatal Abstinence Syndrome

Christine Perez, PhD, BSN, RN, CEIM

KEYWORDS

- Neonatal opioid withdrawal syndrome • Neonatal abstinence syndrome
- Nonpharmacological • Eat sleep console • Standardization
- State Perinatal Quality Collaboratives • Quality initiatives
- Family-centered individualized care

KEY POINTS

- In the United States, there is a substantial increase in the use of opioids and substances during pregnancy, negatively affecting newborns and separating families, leading to strains on health care and social systems.
- More than half of newborns with opioid withdrawal may be treated with non-pharmacological measures, reducing the need for pharmacologic treatment and admittance to neonatal intensive care units.
- The Eat Sleep Console care approach provides an individualized family-centered approach versus a medical model of care for neonatal abstinence syndrome/neonatal opioid withdrawal syndrome (NAS/NOWS).
- State Perinatal Quality Collaboratives and single-center quality initiatives with interprofessional collaboration are integral to transitioning the care approach for NAS/NOWS.
- Identifying barriers to family presence at the bedside for NAS/NOWS in birthing hospitals, such as social determinants of health, mental health, and perceived health care provider stigma of birthing and parenting people with substance use, is critical.

INTRODUCTION

In the United States, opioid use in pregnancy increased by 131% from 2010 to 2017.[1] Risk factors for opioid use in pregnancy include (1) non-Hispanic White,[1,2] (2) median age of 25 to 29 years,[1] (3) residing in the lowest quartile of median income, (4) living in rural counties,[1,3] (5) lower unemployment rates,[4] (6) receive no prenatal care or not until the third trimester,[2] (7) tobacco and alcohol use,[2] and (8) higher incidence of mental

NICU Thought Leader Philips, Infant Massage USA, 8800 Lombard Place 1507, San Diego, CA 92122, USA
E-mail address: perezchristine4@gmail.com

Crit Care Nurs Clin N Am 36 (2024) 223–233
https://doi.org/10.1016/j.cnc.2023.11.005
0899-5885/24/© 2023 Elsevier Inc. All rights reserved.

health illness.[2,5,6] The use of amphetamines and opioids in pregnancy increases the maternal risk for adult respiratory distress syndrome and preterm labor. In addition, amphetamines in pregnancy increase the risk of severe maternal morbidity and mortality, including heart failure, eclampsia, and two times the incidence of preeclampsia.[3] The Centers for Disease Control and Prevention[7] defines neonatal abstinence syndrome (NAS) as newborn withdrawal from substance exposure in utero before birth, noting in utero exposure and withdrawal of opioids in the first 28 days of life is known as neonatal opioid withdrawal syndrome (NOWS) and is a subset of NAS. In 2016, the median length of stay for babies with NAS was 15.9 days, and average hospital costs were $22,552,[8] resulting in triple the costs of hospital charges to $2.5 billion for NAS[9] with greater than 80% of costs covered by Medicaid.[8,10]

A lack of standardization for NAS/NOWS leads to an increase in admissions into neonatal intensive care units (NICUs).[11,12] From 2004 to 2013, rates of NAS admission to NICUs had an increase of six to seven times from 7 to 27 cases per 1000 admissions.[13] Separation of families often occurs with babies diagnosed with NAS, costing $1.6 to 1.9 billion nationally for foster care.[14] Health care providers seek guidance from public health officials in standardizing care for NAS/NOWS to decrease health care expenditures while supporting families. The public health response is non-pharmacological care beginning at birth to prevent separation and unnecessary admissions into NICUs.[15] As a result, there is a paradigm shift in care from a medical model of care with a pharmacologic focus to a family-centered, non-pharmacological individualized approach for NAS/NOWS.

Prevalence and Long-Term Implications of Neonatal Abstinence Syndrome/Neonatal Opioid Withdrawal Syndrome

In the United States, data from 2017 indicate that the prevalence of NAS varies from state to state, from 1.3 to 53.5 per 1000 births, with the highest incidence in West Virginia.[1] States with punitive policies for substance use in pregnancy[4] and areas with a shortage of mental health services[16] further increase the incidence of NAS.[4,16] Prenatal exposure to opioids with a NOWS diagnosis is associated with a mortality rate of 6 per 1000 live births, with a significant increase in mortality of 20 per 1000 live births for opioid exposure without a NOWS diagnosis.[6] Newborns with NAS/NOWS mean gestational age at birth are 38.4 weeks,[1,4] with a higher risk in males.[4,9,17]

NAS/NOWS result in an increase in health care expenditures at birth and the first 8 years of childhood, with dehydration and feeding issues as primary diagnoses within the first month to year of life.[2] The number of inpatient readmissions with a history of NOWS is quadrupled,[18] and there are higher rates of emergency department and outpatient visits.[18,19] NOWS is associated with an increased risk for sensory, language, and developmental delays,[20] as well as behavior, emotional, and speech disorders.[21] In school years, children with a history of NOWS are more likely to require therapy assistance in the school setting.[22] Pennsylvania reported a cost of $506, 523 annually for special education related to these patients,[23] highlighting the necessity for initiating therapy services in the postpartum period and promoting early intervention for NAS/NOWS.

Clinical Signs and Symptoms of Neonatal Abstinence Syndrome/Neonatal Opioid Withdrawal Syndrome

Signs of withdrawal in newborns begin within the first 1 to 3 days after birth,[15] and symptoms can persist for weeks and months.[24] Newborn substance withdrawal symptoms impact the central and autonomic nervous systems, gastrointestinal tract, as well as sleep patterns (eg, **Table 1**).

Table 1
Clinical signs neonatal substance withdrawal

Central Nervous System	Gastrointestinal	Sleep Patterns	Autonomic Nervous System
Increased muscle tone[15,25]	Diarrhea[15,25]	Sleep fragmentation (<2–3 after feeding)[25]	Fevers[15,24]
Irritability[15]	Vomiting[15]	Decrease in quiet sleep[26]	Sweating[15,24]
Seizure activity[15]	Feeding difficulties[15,25]	Lower threshold wakefulness[26]	Tachypnea[15,24]
Tremors (disturbed or undisturbed)[25]	Dysrhythmic feeding patterns[15]		Nasal stuffiness[15,24]
Excessive crying[25]	Weight loss[24]		Frequent yawning[15,24]
	Hyperphagia[25]		Sneezing[15,24]
	Feeding intolerance[25]		Respiratory distress[27]

The US Health and Human Services Division[28] identified that there had been no standard clinical definition for NOWS in the last 45 years. This led to a collaboration of experts defining clinical criteria for NOWS to include both in utero exposure to opioids and two of the five clinical signs of substance withdrawal, (1) excessive crying, (2) fragmented sleep, (3) tremors, (4) increased muscle tone, and (5) gastrointestinal dysfunction.[25] Separation from family in NAS/NOWS may also result in symptoms similar to withdrawal,[15] and with a prolonged stay in the NICU, newborns with NAS/NOWS with unmet needs can exhibit learned withdrawal behaviors, resulting in unnecessary pharmacologic treatment that even furthers the infant's hospital stay.[29]

Approach

Traditionally, in the United States, since the 1970s, the Finnegan Neonatal Abstinence Scoring System has been used to assess the severity of withdrawal signs and determine the treatment approach for NAS/NOWS[30]; however, this may result in unnecessary pharmacologic treatment leading to longer hospital stays.[31] The Eat, Sleep, Console (ESC) care approach assesses newborns with NAS/NOWS ability to breastfeed well or eat 1 or more ounces of feeding, sleep undisturbed for 1 hour or longer, and is consolable within 10 minutes when crying.[31] The ESC care approach has significantly reduced newborns with NAS/NOWS hospital length of stay, the necessity for pharmacologic treatment, and admittance into NICU.[31] The Yale New Haven Children's Hospital (YHNC) using the ESC approach reduced pharmacologic treatment from 62% to 12%:[31] another hospital reported a 65% reduction in NICU admissions.[32] The reduction in length of stays with the ESC approach varied from 7 to 14 days,[31,33,34] with a median length of stay (LOS) with ESC of 5.9 days.[31,35] The Washington Department of Health announced the state would require hospitals to use the ESC model of care for substance-exposed infants as best practice transitioning away from pharmacologic and NICU admission approaches.[36]

Pharmacologic Treatment

Nationally, there is a lack of standardized pharmacologic treatment for NAS/NOWS. Despite the recommendation for non-pharmacological interventions as the first line of treatment, there has been an increase in pharmacologic treatment for NAS from 74% in 2004 to 87% in 2013.[13] Less than 60% of 145 birthing hospitals surveyed in California reported having a written protocol for initiating and discontinuing pharmacologic treatment, whereas less than 50% have escalation and weaning protocols in place.[30] Oral morphine and methadone are the most common first line medications for pharmacologic treatment for NAS.[30] Dosage and frequency varies by organization, noting symptom-based dosing requires more adjunctive treatment in comparison to weight-based dosing with morphine.[37] Utilization of the ESC approach significantly decreases the use of pharmacologic treatment, with a reported 84% decrease in the use of morphine for methadone-exposed infants.[38] Second line adjunctive pharmacologic treatments for NAS/NOWS include phenobarbital and clonidine.[15,39] Blood pressure monitoring is necessary for the use of clonidine due to the risk of hypotension and hypertension.[9] The mean morphine treatment duration was significantly longer with clonidine (34.4 days, SD = 10.6) compared with phenobarbital (25.5 days, SD = 7.3, p = .026). The clonidine group also had higher inpatient adjunctive days and length of stay compared with phenobarbital.[39] Parental presence at the bedside also decreases the need for pharmacologic treatment[40] and improves the transition to a family-centered approach.

Non-pharmacological treatment

The ACT NOW Clinical Practice Survey of 28 states and 54 centers identified that 20% of NICU and non-ICU settings lacked non-pharmacological policies, highlighting the necessity to standardize care for babies diagnosed with NAS/NOWS.[41] Non-pharmacological interventions for NAS/NOWS fall into the following categories: (1) nurturing environment, (2) supporting families, (3) comfort measures, (4) feeding strategies, and (5) therapeutic modalities. Non-pharmacological care for NOWS begins with a nurturing environment with a preferred design of private rooms,[42,43] providing a low-stimulation environment[42,44] with dim lighting and reduced loud noises,[45–47] utilizing soft voices,[48] and maintaining a stable room temperature.[49] Supporting family-centered care for babies with NAS/NOWS includes rooming-in to help promote zero separation.[43] It also provides opportunities for parental care participation and engagement, including talking, reading, and singing to the baby.[29] All of these, as well as skin-to-skin contact helps to promote bonding and attachment, while at the same time increasing parental empowerment and confidence.[44,49] to promote bonding and attachment while increasing parental empowerment and confidence. Non-pharmacological comfort measures such as swings with vertical rocking,[29] holding,[48] containment holds,[29] swaddling,[42,44] swaddle bathing,[29] and offering cuddlers when the family is not present, all may reduce the severity of withdrawal in the baby. Feeding strategies that may reduce the severity of withdrawal symptoms for NAS/NOWS infants includes breastfeeding (the preferred method of feeding)[47,48] non-nutritive sucking,[42,44] as well as providing small, frequent, on-demand, and high caloric feedings.[29,42,44] Therapeutic modalities for NAS/NOWS include hydrotherapy, performing range of motion interventions, providing infant massage, aromatherapy, music therapy, specifically with quiet rhythms and pitch with only 2 to 3 chords, the use of lullabies or nursery rhymes, or providing white noise, (precisely the shushing sound).[29] During the acute withdrawal phase, newborns with NAS/NOWS experience difficulty with self-regulation. A cue-based, individualized, non-pharmacological approach with modifications helps the baby self-regulate.[29] Parents with substance use disorder may also be in withdrawal,[29] and may have difficulty self-regulating and understanding their babies' cues.[29] Providing families with education, support, and a toolbox of non-pharmacological interventions (eg, **Table 2**) assists in establishing a routine in the hospital for a smoother transition to home.

Table 2
Non-pharmacological toolbox neonatal abstinence syndrome/neonatal opioid withdrawal syndrome

Nurturing Environment	Supporting Families	Comfort	Feeding Strategies	Therapeutic Modalities
Private rooms (preferred)[42,43]	Rooming-in[43]	Swing (vertical rocking)[29]	Breastfeeding[47,48]	Hydrotherapy[29]
Low-stimulation environment[42,44]	Zero-separation[29]	Carriers[29]	On-demand feeding[29]	Music therapy (quiet rhythm and pitch, lullabies, nursery rhymes, 2–3 chords)[29]
Reduction of lighting and noise[45,47]	Talking to baby[29]	Containment holds[29]	Small frequent feeding[42]	White noise: Shushing sound[29]
Quiet calm environment[47]	Reading to baby[29]	Vertical rocking[29]	Nonnutritive suck[42,44]	Range of motion
Dim lighting[45,47]	Singing to baby[29]	Holding[48]	High-calorie feeds[44]	Infant massage[29]
Soft voices[48]	Skin-to-skin[44,49]	Swaddling[42,44]		Aromatherapy[29]
Stable room temperature[49]	Parental engagement[29]	Swaddle Bathing[29]		
	Care participation[29]	Cuddler program (when family not present)[29]		

Implementation and standardization

State Perinatal Quality Collaboratives (SPQCs) are a network of perinatal health care providers and public health officials collaborating through quality initiatives (QIs) to develop standardized, evidence-based practices for NAS/NOWS.[42] SPQCs have successfully reduced pharmacologic treatment and length of hospital stays in babies with NAS/NOWS. The Ohio Perinatal Quality Collaborative promoted standardized treatment for NOWS throughout 54 facilities by initiating a state-level quality initiative that, reduced the length of stay by 1.3 days and treatments by 1.4 days.[50] Single-Center Quality Initiatives (SCQIs) have been instrumental in transitioning the care approach for NAS/NOWS. The YNHC, in 2010, began a QI using the plan-do-study-act (PDSA) methodology to standardize non-pharmacological care for babies with NAS/NOWS.[38] Primary approaches were staff education on non-pharmacological care, admittance of NAS/NOWS to an inpatient unit versus the NICU, administration of pharmacologic treatment as needed versus a standard routine treatment, and empowering parents all of which resulted in a reduction in length of stay from 22.4 days to 5.9 days, and a decrease in costs from $44,824 to $10, 289,[38] highlighting the benefits of transitioning the care approach for NAS/NOWS.

The initial step to initiate a QI for the transition in care approach for NAS/NOWS is to develop an interprofessional team that includes numerous key stakeholders, including (1) neonatology, (2) nursing staff, NICU leadership including directors, managers, and educators, newborn nursery staff, and pediatric staff, (3) therapy services, (4) case managers, (5) child life therapy, (6) developmental specialists, (7) social worker, (8) dietician, (9) family advocate, and (10) the health department including guidance from SPQCs.[29] Core teams assist in driving culture change and obtaining buy-in from health care providers.[29] The core team develops a meeting cadence to develop policies, protocols, guidelines, and staff and family education while identifying barriers and facilitators to implementation and standardization.[29] The PDSA methodology assists in facilitating change[35] and incorporates modifications to the process, such as the need for additional resources and staffing workflows.[29] Obtaining feedback from families and staff on the new care approach for NAS/NOWS provides an opportunity to identify barriers and facilitators to embedding new practices into workflow and standardizing care.[29] Education for staff on non-pharmacological care for NAS/NOWS should be all-inclusive for any team member who works with this population and should be continual.[29] Family education for non-pharmacological interventions for NAS/NOWS should be 1:1 training with return demonstrations, and handouts should be in both written and digital formats to facilitate a smooth transition home.[29]

COMPLICATIONS/CONCERNS

SPQCs have successfully reduced pharmacologic treatment for NAS/NOWS; however, over time, there is less than 60% adherence to non-pharmacological measures.[50] Organizational structure may also create barriers to SCQI transitioning the care approach for NAS/NOWS, noting implementation process times are variable from 1 to 6 years.[29] Social determinants of health may create barriers for families of newborns with NAS/NOWS to be at the bedside, including lack of childcare, transportation, and/ or family support.[29] In a retrospective study from 2018 to 2020, a regional center with a geographically dispersed population and families driving 2 or more hours to reach the NICU, 41% of the evaluations showed that no families were present, and results indicated the ESC care approach did not decrease the length of stay or pharmacologic treatment.[51,52] Staffing workflows can also be a barrier to the ESC approach if families are absent,[29] as NAS/NOWS require more nursing time for care.[53] Health care provider stigma of pregnant and parenting individuals with opioid use disorder can also create a barrier to parental presence for NAS/NOWS,[29] as they are less likely to access services and treatment if there is a perception of stigma.[54]

Parental barriers to providing non-pharmacological interventions for newborns with NAS/NOWS include a lack of knowledge and apprehension of withdrawal symptoms, fearfulness, and the ability to self-regulate and understand their babies' cues.[29] Because of the rates of readmission for infants with NAS/NOWS, are frequently dehydration and feeding difficulties, it is critical to link families with community resources, including postpartum home visitation programs. In addition, long-term developmental complications for babies with NAS/NOWS demonstrates the need for therapy services beginning in birthing hospitals[29] as well as continued early intervention services in the community.[55]

FUTURE DIRECTIONS

Hospitals and public health officials must continue to collaborate to transition the care approach for babies with NAS/NOWS from a medical model of care to a family-centered, individualized, non-pharmacological approach to care. Public health policies must address the variability in care for babies with NAS/NOWS in hospital settings and their access to early intervention. There needs to be an increase in community awareness of the negative impact of the use of substances in pregnancy to newborns, including withdrawal symptoms and long-term implications. Education for healthcare providers on NAS/NOWS patients as well as pregnant and parenting individuals with substance use disorder is warranted to decrease the stigma associated with substance abuse which creates a barrier to providing high-quality care. Addressing social determinants of health is also critical to ensure equitable care for infants with NAS/NOWS and their families.

In summary, addressing NAS/NOWS requires a multifaceted approach involving collaboration between hospitals, public health officials, health care providers, communities, and various levels of government. This approach should prioritize the well-being of newborns with NAS/NOWS and their families, provide evidence-based care while reducing stigmas and ensure equitable access to care. Further research on NAS/NOWS, including long-term implications of the ESC care approach and outcomes of newborns with substance exposure in utero without a diagnosis of NAS/NOWS, will provide guidance for improving care and outcomes in the future.

CLINICS CARE POINTS

- Develop neonatal abstinence syndrome/neonatal opioid withdrawal syndrome (NAS/NOWS) cross-disciplinary committee with interprofessional team members (eg, certified neonatal therapists, neonatologists, pediatricians, neonatal intensive care unit [NICU] and postpartum nursing staff, nursing leadership, educators, social workers, mental health providers, developmental specialists, dieticians, child life specialists, and lactation consultants) and establish a meeting cadence.

- Conduct clinical benchmarking of facilities using family-centered individualized non-pharmacological care as the primary care approach for NAS/NOWS.

- Initiate a quality initiative project for NAS/NOWS using plan-do-study-act methodology.

- Collaborate with the State Perinatal Quality Collaboratives.[51]

- Conduct a baseline assessment of nursing staffing workflows and identify gaps for implementing the ESC approach; develop a staffing committee before implementation as needed.
- Identify unit-specific barriers to family presence, including social determinants of health and parental mental health.
- Develop and obtain approvals for evidence-based policies and protocols for NAS/NOWS, including pharmacologic and non-pharmacological interventions.
- Identify additional funding and staffing resources needed.
- Review admission order sets in units with NAS/NOWS admissions, including postpartum, pediatrics, and NICU, and verify the inclusion of automatic orders for therapy and social services.
- Review pharmacologic treatment guidelines for NAS/NOWS to ensure inclusion of initiation, escalation, weaning, and discontinuation, as well as consider weight-based dosing versus symptoms dosing, noting that clonidine requires blood pressure monitoring.
- Develop and implement electronic medical record (EMR) smart phrases for non-pharmacological care interventions (eg, see **Table 2**).
- Review reimbursement coding practices for NAS/NOWS.
- Develop an education plan for all staff interacting with NAS/NOWS patients and families.
- Promote family-centered care for NAS/NOWS by providing resources for parents to be present at the bedside and initiate education and inclusion on non-pharmacological care interventions beginning on admission to support parental engagement, empowerment, and confidence.
- Resources for families should be in written and digital formats (handouts, QR codes, digital platforms) and establish a routine in the hospital.
- Conduct interdisciplinary rounds to identify any modifications needed in policy/procedures or resources for NAS/NOWS and individualized plan of care.
- Develop audits to monitor adherence to non-pharmacological interventions for NAS/NOWS.
- Provide feedback opportunities from NICU staff and families on new policies/protocols and care for NAS/NOWS (eg, survey, 1:1 bedside feedback).
- Develop a cadence for the review of policies and procedures for infants with NAS/NOWS.
- Before discharge, link families to community resources, including postpartum home visitation programs, mental health services, and early intervention programs.
- Post-discharge monitoring should assess weight gain/growth, feeding difficulties, achievement of developmental milestones, infant–parent attachment, and parental mental health.

DISCLOSURE

The author has no commercial or financial conflicts of interest and did not receive funding for this article.

REFERENCES

1. Hirai AH, Ko JY, Owens PL, et al. Neonatal abstinence syndrome and maternal opioid-related diagnoses in the US, 2010-2017. JAMA 2021;325(2):146–55.
2. Ko JY, Wolicki S, Barfield WD, et al. CDC grand rounds: public health strategies to prevent neonatal abstinence syndrome. MMWR (Morb Mortal Wkly Rep) 2017;66(9):242.

3. Admon LK, Bart G, Kozhimannil KB, et al. Amphetamine-and opioid-affected births: incidence, outcomes, and costs, United States, 2004–2015. Am J Public Health 2019;109(1):148–54.

4. Faherty LJ, Stein BD, Terplan M. Consensus guidelines and state policies: the gap between principle and practice at the intersection of substance use and pregnancy. Am J Obstet Gynecol MFM 2020;2(3):e100137.

5. Corr TE, Hollenbeak CS. The economic burden of neonatal abstinence syndrome in the United States. J Addict 2017;112(9):1590–9.

6. Leyenaar JK, Schaefer AP, Wasserman JR, et al. Infant mortality associated with prenatal opioid exposure. JAMA Pediatr 2021;175(7):706–14.

7. Center for Disease Control and Prevention. About opioid use in pregnancy. cdc.gov. https://www.cdc.gov/pregnancy/opioids/basics.html Accessed on October 1, 2023.

8. Strahan AE, Guy GP, Bohm M, et al. Neonatal abstinence syndrome incidence and health care costs in the United States, 2016. JAMA Pediatr 2020;174(2):200–2.

9. Ramphul K, Mejias SG, Joynauth J. An update on the burden of neonatal abstinence syndrome in the United States. Hosp Pediatr 2020;10(2):181–4.

10. Umer A, Lilly C, Hamilton C, et al. Disparities in neonatal abstinence syndrome and health insurance status: a statewide study using non–claims real-time surveillance data. Paediatr Perinat Epidemiol 2021;35(3):330–8.

11. Howard MB, Schiff DM, Penwill N, et al. Impact of parental presence at infants' bedside on neonatal abstinence syndrome. Hosp Pediatr 2017;7(2):63–9.

12. Wachman EM, Schiff DM, Silverstein M. Neonatal abstinence syndrome: advances in diagnosis and treatment. JAMA 2018;319(13):1362–74.

13. Tolia VN, Patrick SW, Bennett MM, et al. Increasing incidence of neonatal abstinence syndrome in US neonatal ICUs. NEJM 2015;372(22):2118–26.

14. Crowley DM, Connell CM, Jones D, et al. Considering the child welfare system burden from opioid misuse: research priorities for estimating public costs. AJMC 2019;25(13):S256–63.

15. Patrick SW, Barfield WD, Poindexter BB, et al. Neonatal opioid withdrawal syndrome. An Pediatr 2020;146(5). https://doi.org/10.1542/peds.2020-029074. e2020029074.

16. Patrick SW, Frank RG, McNeer E, et al. Improving the child welfare system to respond to the needs of substance-exposed infants. Hosp Pediatr 2019;9(8):651–4.

17. Leech AA, Cooper WO, McNeer E, et al. Neonatal abstinence syndrome in the United States, 2004–16: an examination of neonatal abstinence syndrome trends and incidence patterns across US census regions in the period 2004–16. Health Aff 2020;39(5):764–7.

18. Liu G, Kong L, Leslie DL, et al. A longitudinal healthcare use profile of children with a history of neonatal abstinence syndrome. J Pediatr 2019;204:111–7.

19. Hwang SS, Weikel B, Adams J, et al. The Colorado Hospitals Substance Exposed Newborn Quality Improvement Collaborative: standardization of care for opioid-exposed newborns shortens length of stay and reduces the number of infants requiring opiate therapy. Hosp Pediatr 2020;10(9):783–91.

20. Fucile S, Gallant H, Patel A. Developmental outcomes of children born with neonatal abstinence syndrome (NAS): a scoping review. Phys Occup Ther Pediatr 2020;41(1):85–98.

21. Hall ES, McAllister JM, Wexelblatt SL. Developmental disorders and medical complications among infants with subclinical intrauterine opioid exposures. PHM 2019;22(1):19–24.

22. Fill MMA, Miller AM, Wilkinson RH, et al. Educational disabilities among children born with neonatal abstinence syndrome. An Pediatr 2018;142(3):e20180562.
23. Morgan PL, Wang Y. The opioid epidemic, neonatal abstinence syndrome, and estimated costs for special education services. AJMC 2019;25(13 Suppl): S264–9.
24. Reddy UM, Davis JM, Ren Z, et al. Opioid use in pregnancy, neonatal abstinence syndrome, and childhood outcomes: executive summary of a joint workshop by the Eunice Kennedy Shriver national institute of child health and human development, American congress of obstetricians and gynecologists, American academy of pediatrics, society for maternal-fetal medicine, centers for Disease Control and prevention, and the march of dimes foundation. OBGYN 2017; 130(1):10.
25. Jilani SM, Jones HE, Grossman M, et al. Standardizing the clinical definition of opioid withdrawal in the neonate. J Pediatr 2022;243:33–9.
26. Barbeau DY, Weiss MD. Sleep disturbances in newborns. Children 2017; 4(10):90.
27. Hussaini KS, Saavedra LFG. Neonatal abstinence syndrome (NAS) in southwestern border states: examining trends, population correlates, and implications for policy. Matern Child Health J 2018;22(9):1352–9.
28. United States Department of Health and Human Services (2022, January 31). HHS announces a standard clinical definition for opioid withdrawal in infants. https://www.hhs.gov/about/news/2022/01/31/hhs-announces-standard-clinical-definition-for-opioid-withdrawal-in-infants.html.
29. Perez C. Exploring infant massage as standard nonpharmacological treatment for neonatal opioid withdrawal syndrome. PQDT 2022 (2709971970). Available at: https://www.proquest.com/dissertations-theses/exploring-infant-massage-as-standard/docview/2709971970/se-2. Accessed on October 1, 2023.
30. Clemans-Cope L, Holla N, Lee HC, et al. Neonatal abstinence syndrome management in California birth hospitals: results of a statewide survey. Am J Perinatol 2020;40(3):463–72.
31. Grossman MR, Lipshaw MJ, Osborn RR, et al. A novel approach to assessing infants with neonatal abstinence syndrome. Hosp Pediatr 2018;8(1):1–6.
32. Spence K, Boedeker R, Harhausen M, et al. Avoiding NICU transfers for newborns with neonatal opioid withdrawal syndrome (NOWS): a quality improvement initiative to manage NOWS on the mother-baby unit. JAM 2020;14(5):401–8.
33. Achilles JS, Castaneda-Lovato J. A quality improvement initiative to improve the care of infants born exposed to opioids by implementing the eat, sleep, console assessment tool. Hosp Pediatr 2019;9(8):624–31.
34. Young LW, Ounpraseuth ST, Merhar SL, et al. Eat, sleep, console approach or usual care for Neonatal Opioid Withdrawal. N Engl J Med 2023;388:2326–37.
35. Dodds D, Koch K, Buitrago-Mogollon T, et al. Successful implementation of the eat sleep console model of care for infants with NAS in a community hospital. Hosp Pediatr 2019;9(8):632–8.
36. Washinton State Department of Health. State agencies announce changes in policy and best practices for infants and parents affected by substance use at birth. doh.wa.gov. https://doh.wa.gov/newsroom/state-agencies-announce-changes-policy-and-best-practices-infants-and-parents-affected-substance-use. Accessed on October 8, 2023.
37. Harris JB, Holmes AP. Comparison of two morphine dosing strategies in the management of Neonatal Abstinence Syndrome. JPTT 2022;27(2):151–6.

38. Grossman MR, Berkwitt AK, Osborn RR, et al. An initiative to improve the quality of care of infants with neonatal abstinence syndrome. An Pediatr 2017;139(6). e20163360.
39. Brusseau C, Burnette T, Heidel RE. Clonidine versus phenobarbital as adjunctive therapy for neonatal abstinence syndrome. J Perinatol 2020;40(7):1050–5.
40. Scott LF, Guilfoy V, Duwve JM, et al. Factors associated with the need for pharmacological management of neonatal opioid withdrawal syndrome. Advan Neonatal Care 2020;20(5):364–73.
41. Snowden JN, Akshatha A, Annett RD, et al. The ACT NOW clinical practice survey: gaps in the care of infants with neonatal opioid withdrawal syndrome. Hosp Pediatr 2019;9(8):585–92.
42. Krans EE, Patrick SW. Opioid use disorder in pregnancy: health policy and practice in the midst of an epidemic. OGYN 2016;128(1):4–10.
43. Avram CM, Yieh L, Dukhovny D, et al. A cost-effectiveness analysis of rooming-in and breastfeeding in neonatal opioid withdrawal. Am. J. Perinat 2020;37(01):001–7.
44. Kurup U, Merchant N. Neonatal abstinence syndrome: management and current concepts. PCH 2020;31(1):24–31.
45. Mangat AK, Schmölzer GM, Kraft WK. Pharmacological and non-pharmacological treatments for the neonatal abstinence syndrome (NAS). Semin Fetal Neonatal Med 2019;24(2):133–41.
46. Singleton R, Slaunwhite A, Herrick M, et al. Research and policy priorities for addressing prenatal exposure to opioids in Alaska. Int J Circumpolar Health 2019; 78(1):e1599275.
47. Ryan G, Dooley J, Gerber Finn L, et al. Nonpharmacological management of neonatal abstinence syndrome: a review of the literature. J Matern Fetal Neonatal Med 2019;32(10):1735–40.
48. Sander A, Henderson C, Metz G, et al. Specialized care of women and newborns affected by opioids with a CORE team of nurses. Nur Womens Health 2018;22(4): 327–31.
49. Oostlander SA, Falla JA, Dow K, et al. Occupational therapy management strategies for infants with neonatal abstinence syndrome: scoping review. Occup Ther Health Care 2019;33(2):197–226.
50. Walsh MC, Crowley M, Wexelblatt S, et al. Ohio Perinatal Quality Collaborative improves care of neonatal narcotic abstinence syndrome. An Pediatr 2018;141(4). https://doi.org/10.1542/peds.2017-0900. e20170900.
51. Amin A, Frazie M, Thompson S, et al. Assessing the Eat, Sleep, Console model for neonatal abstinence syndrome management at a regional referral center. J Perinatol 2023;43:916–22.
52. Center for Disease Control and Prevention. State perinatal quality collaboritives.cdc.gov. https://www.cdc.gov/reproductivehealth/maternalinfanthealth/pqc-states.html. Accessed October 9, 2023.
53. Smith JG, Rogowski JA, Schoenauer KM, et al. Infants in drug withdrawal: a national description of nurse workload, infant acuity, and parental needs. J Perinat Neonatal Nurs 2018;32(1):72–9.
54. Crawford AD, McGlothen-Bell K, Recto P, et al. Stigmatization of pregnant individuals with opioid use disorder. Women's Health Rep 2022;3(1):172–9.
55. Ohio Department of Developmental Disabilities. Neonatal abstinence syndrome.dodd.ohio.gov, https://dodd.ohio.gov/your-family/all-family-resources/resource-neonatal-abstinence-syndrome-ei. Accessed October 10, 2023.

Neonatal Abstinence Syndrome/Neonatal Opioid Withdrawal Syndrome

An Ecological View of Non-Pharmacologic Interventions for Feeding Success

Ashlea D. Cardin, OTD, OTR/L, BCP, CNT

KEYWORDS

- Neonatal abstinence • Withdrawal • Feeding
- Ecology of Human Performance model

KEY POINTS

- NAS/NOWS is known to disrupt dyadic infant–caregiver feeding development and success.
- Non-pharmacologic interventions to promote feeding success may be categorized into Establish/Restore, Alter, Adapt/Modify, Prevent, and Create approaches.
- The safety and efficacy of non-pharmacologic interventions need further investigation to provide clear guidelines for clinical practice.

INTRODUCTION

As opioid use continues to climb in the United States and globally,[1–3] the number of infants exposed prenatally to both licit and illicit substances and subsequently diagnosed with neonatal abstinence syndrome (NAS) or neonatal opioid withdrawal syndrome (NOWS) has also increased. According to the Centers for Disease Control and Prevention, 59 newborns—more than one infant every 24 minutes—are diagnosed every day.[4] In the United States, NAS/NOWS is a recognized public health crisis with notable state-level and regional variation. Nationwide, NAS hospitalizations have grown nearly eightfold[5] and increased significantly to 7.3 infants per 1000 birth hospitalizations[6] with the highest rates of NAS occurring in the Midwest and in rural areas.[5–9]

According to Anbalagan and Mendez,[10] NAS is a "spectrum of clinical manifestations seen in neonates due to withdrawal from intrauterine drug exposure."[(p1)]

Missouri State University, 901 S. National Avenue, OCHS 203H, Springfield, MO 65897, USA
E-mail address: ashleacardin@missouristate.edu

Crit Care Nurs Clin N Am 36 (2024) 235–249
https://doi.org/10.1016/j.cnc.2023.11.010
0899-5885/24/© 2024 Elsevier Inc. All rights reserved.

NOWS is considered an opioid-specific subset of NAS[11] which "presents with a variety of dysregulated physiologic and behavioral reactions that appear after discontinuation of exposure to exogenous opioids at birth."[12(para 2)] Polydrug exposure is common in NAS/NOWS, but recent trends demonstrate increasingly higher incidences of opioid use among pregnant women. As such, NOWS is a clinical diagnosis that describes a "constellation of symptoms" that results from the abrupt discontinuation of chronic exposure to opioid use in pregnancy.[10(p9)]

The expression of NAS/NOWS symptoms differs in severity, and it is unclear what causes the variation or why premature infants, for example, are less likely to express severe symptoms when compared with term infants.[10] It has been posited that expressive inconsistencies may arise due to genetic and epigenetic profiles,[13,14] maternal history, and polydrug exposure, including that of prescribed medication and nicotine.[15,16] Infants diagnosed with NAS/NOWS may demonstrate mild to severe disturbances in their central nervous system, which leads to negative physiologic responses including exaggerated Moro reflex, changes in skin color, and breathing and digestive disturbances.[17–19] Withdrawal symptoms, including excessive or high-pitched crying, agitation, fever or temperature instability, tremors, poor quality and duration of sleep, altered sleep-wake cycles, sweating, vomiting, diarrhea, perianal skin breakdown, weight loss, seizures, yawning, sneezing, and increased muscle tone, may subsequently impact an infant's ability to effectively participate in activities such as feeding.[17,20–22]

PHARMACOLOGIC AND NON-PHARMACOLOGIC SYMPTOM MANAGEMENT

Evidence guiding pharmacologic intervention for infants born with a physiologic dependence on opioids and/or other psychotropic drugs remains unstandardized. This is affirmed by the work of Yen and colleagues,[14] who report hospital-based practice variation as a key challenge in the management of NAS/NOWS. Patrick and Lorch[5] reported that "it is apparent that 2[sic] decades into the present opioid crisis … one of our nation's most vulnerable populations is receiving highly variable care, resulting in disparate outcomes.[(p e2020028340)] This is concerning, as Wu and Carre[23] report that 27% to 91% of infants with NAS will require pharmacologic intervention. Although an extensive review of pharmacologic treatment is beyond the scope of this article, standardized pharmacologic symptom management is currently under study[24,25] with multiple federal initiatives aimed at addressing knowledge gaps.[26]

From an evidentiary standpoint, a growing number of explanatory and exploratory studies are beginning to pair or "bundle" pharmacologic medical treatment with non-pharmacologic interventions to manage NAS/NOWS symptoms,[5,19,23,27–31] and research has expanded to include interprofessional non-pharmacologic therapeutic approaches and interventions.[32,33] Although specific interventions vary,[34] the use of non-pharmacologic care and treatment approaches is becoming standard practice in hospital systems around the globe.[1,35] As "the goal of non-pharmacological treatment is to assist the self-organization of the neonate and support neuro-maturation,"[10(p16)], non-pharmacologic interventions may be deployed to reduce or eliminate the need for replacement opioids while targeting outcomes such as altered developmental trajectories,[19] duration of pharmacologic intervention, hospital length of stay,[36] and feeding dysfunction.

NEONATAL ABSTINENCE SYNDROME/NEONATAL OPIOID WITHDRAWAL SYNDROME AND FEEDING

For infants hospitalized with NAS/NOWS, signs of withdrawal typically begin within the first few days of life,[10,19] considered a critical period for early feeding skill establishment, nourishment, parent–infant attachment, and co-occupational feeding success.[37] A pivotal early developmental milestone for infants, feeding is a highly complex and purposeful activity that necessitates infants have adequate motor, processing, and social interaction performance skills, sensory modulation capability, and typically functioning body systems in coordination with an appropriate behavioral state.[38–42] According to Maguire and colleagues,[17] feeding sessions are frequently interrupted by periods of fussing in infants with NAS, often resulting in inadequate nutrition. Velez and colleagues[19] refer to this state of physiologic intolerance and hyperarousal as "outside a window of tolerance,"[(p. 9)] wherein the infant experiencing withdrawal may not be able to feed when hungry, may experience feeding dysfunction and non-restful sleep, and may be unable to engage during feeding visually or socially.

Although the type and severity of withdrawal symptoms and feeding competency vary, infants diagnosed with NAS/NOWS may present with poor state control,[17] gastrointestinal anomalies, swallow dysfunction, sucking difficulties, and hyper-rooting. They may also demonstrate persistent feeding difficulties such as esophageal dysmotility[43]; are 181% more likely to be hospitalized for feeding dysregulation[8]; may experience aberrant early growth, lower birth weights, and disorganized feeding behaviors and decreased oral intake[8,44]; may experience prolonged or delayed hospitalization due to feeding difficulty American Academy of Pediatrics, 2008[40,41,43,45,46]; may overeat to soothe or demonstrate continued feeding difficulty post-hospitalization[32,47–49]; may demonstrate prolonged suck bursts with fewer pauses, increased arousal, and more episodes of spit up or food refusal at developmental follow-up[47]; and may be predisposed to metabolic syndrome in adulthood.[44]

Although the feeding challenges faced by infants experiencing withdrawal are numerous, the infant *per se* is not the sole determiner of feeding success. Dyadic feeding interactions shape each bottle or breastfeeding moment. The adult caregiver's read and response interpretation of infant behavioral cues can determine the shape, pace, and feel of the feeding event.[12,37] As such, infant feeding is known to be "nuanced and influenced by the culture and environment…and by the adults within that environment."[37(p1)] Consideration of feeding as a transactional and ecologically embedded activity suggests that feeding success extends beyond the individual skill and stability of the infant, to include the contextually situated attitudes, culture, resources, and capacity of the professional and familial caregivers surrounding the infant. Dunn[50] posited that "the interaction between person and environment affects behavior and performance, and that performance cannot be understood outside of context."[(p598)] In the presence of a medical diagnosis known to disrupt the infant–caregiver dyad, feeding becomes ever more challenging when considering the universe of personal and environmental variables contributing to—or limiting—feeding success.

AN ECOLOGICAL VIEW OF INFANT FEEDING

Bottle- or breastfeeding is considered a meaningful activity that is shared between the infant and parent or caregiver and shaped by the contextual environment.[37] As such, critical care providers may benefit from a focused, structured examination of disordered feeding experiences within a medical context, with the intent to enhance professional reasoning and inform their selection of subsequent non-pharmacologic interventions. This structure can be provided using the Ecology of Human Performance (EHP) model developed by occupational therapist Winnie Dunn.[50,51] Dunn and her colleagues deliberately developed the EHP model for use beyond occupational therapy; the intent was that EHP could be used by any interprofessional health care provider wishing to support their patients' performance in meaningful activities, such as feeding. As the model is translatable across health care disciplines and medical settings, it is an appropriate choice to examine the multifaceted nature of feeding infants diagnosed with NAS/NOWS.

The core constructs of EHP include an examination of personal, contextual, and task-related factors that interact to either support (or hinder) successful performance in a given task. For example, if critical care providers used the EHP model to guide their reasoning and selection of an appropriate intervention to support feeding success, they would evaluate the following: the infant *and* the parent's (or professional caregiver's) unique abilities, experiences, values, and skills (*person factors*); the behaviors and roles involved in feeding an infant experiencing withdrawal (*task factors*); the enabling—or restrictive—temporal and environmental conditions surrounding the feeding dyad (*context factors*); and finally, the result of the interaction between person, context, and task factors supporting successful feeding performance (*task accomplishment*).

According to Dunn,[51] there are seven steps that health care professionals should take to (1) ensure proper attention is paid to each aspect of human performance and (2) select an appropriate intervention to address performance difficulties or incongruencies. Application of the steps within a NAS/NOWS feeding scenario would require the professional caregiver to:

1. *Determine the dyad's wants, needs, and priorities.* Recognize that "dyad" is defined as a feeding unit of two persons and includes variations such as the infant–mother, infant–parent, infant's family–caregiver, or infant–professional caregiver dyad. Reflect on what the infant may consider "most important" or of high priority,[51(p220)] and what the adult considers most important at the time of feeding.
2. *Analyze the priorities.* Understand the skill requirements of demands on both persons in the feeding dyad. Acknowledge that these may be very different, thus necessitating an individualized response to bring the dyad into feeding goal alignment.
3. *Evaluate the feeding performance.* Which activities, behaviors, or role expectations (of each dyad member) contribute to challenges with the feeding performance?
4. *Evaluate the context* and consider how each dyad's unique situation might affect performance. Context includes each dyad member's age, developmental level, and life stage. Contextual factors influencing feeding also include the physical environment and the objects within the environment; the social environment, including family, friends, and medical professionals interacting with the infant; and the cultural environment, including ethnic, regional, religious, or other shared group norms that shape the dyad's behavior.
5. *Evaluate the personal factors* for both members of the dyad, such as sensorimotor, cognitive, and psychosocial capacity; body structures and functions; personal attributes and abilities; past experiences; and the values and beliefs that contribute to the feeding experience.
6. *Develop prioritized goals* together with the infant and family.
7. *Choose the appropriate intervention strategy(ies)* to support the dyad's feeding success within a medical context: (a) Establish/Restore, (b) Alter, (c) Adapt/Modify, (d) Prevent, and/or (e) Create.

NON-PHARMACOLOGIC INTERVENTIONS TO PROMOTE FEEDING SUCCESS

In a qualitative study by Cardin and colleagues,[37] critical care professionals described positive, successful feeding as infant-driven, wherein the infant shows strong interest in feeding; takes the prescribed volume without stress behaviors or physiologic compromise; remains safe and well-organized; demonstrates efficiency and endurance; sustains engagement; and is self-paced. Participants also recognized their active role in promoting feeding success, stating that professional feeders should be educated in interpreting infant cues and recognizing patterns in infant behaviors, supportive of infant-driven feeding, expertly trained in infant development (especially in light of medical conditions), and "comfortable" [(p4)] when feeding complex infants. Importantly, the critical care providers stated that "skillful feeding reflects a positive experience for both the infant and the feeder." [(p6)] Building on this shared understanding,[45] Pados and Fuller[52] note that multilevel feeding relationships can positively or negatively affect feeding outcomes; when complicated by NAS/NOWS, feeding may be extremely challenging and exceedingly frustrating for both the infant and the familial or professional caregiver. It is in this space that ecologically informed, non-pharmacologic interventions may serve to promote calm and organization within the dyadic feeding interaction.

Evidence examining non-pharmacologic interventions for infants experiencing withdrawal tends to fall within one of two broader categories: interventions that support symptom management which may *indirectly* affect feeding through neurobiological subsystem optimization,[10,11,19,20,33,34,38,53–55] and interventions that *directly* target feeding success in the NAS/NOWS population.[8,17,20,22,23,28,32,34,39,43,45,47,48,56–63]

Assuming a position of critical interpretation and empirical skepticism is necessary, however, as non-pharmacologic intervention research needs to be expanded due to the limitations of existing studies and the lack of comparison data.[64] In their systemic review, Pahl and colleagues[11] found no randomized controlled trials examining the effects of non-pharmacologic intervention on hospital length of stay; however, there are small quasi-experimental and exploratory studies supporting non-pharmacologic intervention to reduce NAS/NOWS outcomes such as length of stay or duration of pharmacologic treatment. Within the growing number of studies supporting direct breastfeeding as an intervention with a host of positive outcomes (attachment, nutrition, maternal emotional health, infant stability, decreased duration of treatment),the Eat, Sleep, Console (ESC) approach is showing promise as a pragmatic and standardized non-pharmacologic intervention that addresses dyadic feeding success.[27,63,65,66] However, additional high-quality evidence is needed.

Regardless of study design or the *direct* versus *indirect* dichotomization, non-pharmacologic interventions for feeding may be reconceptualized using the EHP model and its associated intervention approaches. Doing so provides professional caregivers with a structured view of the types of interventions currently under study or being offered to address feeding challenges in the NAS/NOWS population (**Table 1**). The EHP model is unique in that it includes five different collaborative intervention approaches designed to act on either person, context, or task factors, thereby shifting their influence on feeding performance: Establish/Restore, Alter, Adapt/Modify, Prevent, and Create interventions.

Establish/Restore interventions target person factors. The professional caregiver works to develop the skills, abilities, and intrinsic capabilities of both the infant and the adult feeder (even when that adult feeder is the self) so that feeding performance is maximized. The use of non-pharmacologic interventions may support sensory, autonomic, and motor development in infants with NAS.[19,33] "The quality of the maternal/caregiver responses to the infant's specific needs is affected not only by the severity of the signs of NAS/NOWS but also by the caregiver's own regulatory capacities to respond to the external and internal stressors surrounding the care of the infant during and after hospitalization."[12(p25)]

Table 1
Non-pharmacologic interventions per Ecology of Human Performance approach

EHP Intervention Approach	Target	Interventions
Establish/Restore	Person factors	Interventions should target both individuals in the mother–infant dyad.[19]
	• Infant	• NNS/pacifier use
	• Mother	• Smart bottle technology quantifies suck coordination[32]
	• Family caregivers	• Auricular acupressure sticker feasibility study[67,68]
	• Professional caregivers	• Laser acupuncture[67,69]
	Dyad interaction factors	• Infant massage for pain control, sleep enhancement, stress reduction, and decreased gastrointestinal distress[49,64,70]
		• Prone positioning (while monitored in hospital) or side-lying C-position[10,11]
		• Reiki treatment[64]
		• Swaddling for stimulus reduction[20,60]
		• "Babywearing" reduced infant and caregiver heartrate.[55]
		• Breastfeeding is rarely contraindicated and is now well-established as a non-pharmacologic intervention that may reduce the severity of NAS, length of stay (LOS), and length of pharmacologic treatment (LOT).[20,34,49,56,57]
		• Skin-to-skin holding[48,60]
		• Hand-held containment[20]
		• Holding, swaying, rocking, gentle vertical rocking[20,64,71]
		• Sensory-based interventions provided by occupational therapists to help infants gain the functional skills needed to engage in daily occupations such as feeding.[72]
		• Use of feeding specialists: OT, SLP, lactation consultants[10,32,33,60,72,73]
		• Professional continuing education
Alter	Context (environmental) factors	• Breastfeeding rates are higher with those who room-in[59,60]
	Task factors	• Rooming-in to reduce pharmacotherapy, LOS, mitigate NAS severity, promote breastfeeding success through proximity, and encourage parental presence[28,35,53,59]
		• Use of trained volunteers if family or professionals unavailable[30]
Adapt/Modify	Context (environmental) factors	• Maintaining an environment that has a stable room temperature[33]
	Task factors	• Use of commercially available "automated smart sleeper bed"[30]
		• Mechanical rocking beds, non-oscillating water beds; low-stimulation environments, and vibrotactile stimulation[11,34,74–76]

- Increased caloric intake to mitigate excessive caloric demand of withdrawal[10]
- Formula choice: "The best formula choice for a neonatal abstinence syndrome (NAS) infant is unknown"[56(p1488)]; lactose-free formula did not decrease morphine dose required to treat NAS, LOS, LOT, or daily weight gain.[56,77]
- Maternal breast milk vs formula decreased LOS, LOT, NAS scores.[20,22,78]
- Liu et al[57] found no difference in Finnegan scores between breast fed or bottle-fed infants (either formula or expressed breast milk); further research is needed to determine differences in NAS between "neonates who were breastfed and those who were fed pumped breastmilk or donor milk."[60(p524)]
- Formula flow rate[79]—evaluated preparation type (ready-to-feed vs powder) and formula type (standard vs specialized for reflux). All considered IDDSI thin except for AR ready to feed which was "slightly thick." Reflux formulas were thin but significantly slower than standard formula.
- Caloric dense or thickened feeding may prevent growth failure.[71,80]
- Reduced milk flow rate: most effective bottle type and/or nipple has not been established in this population.[79,81,82]
- Dim lighting/low stimulation[27]
- Environmental modifications to reduce stimulation or promote calm[34,75]
- Aromatherapy[83]
- Frequent, on-demand, small volume feedings[10,11,49,63,65]
- Use of feeding specialists: OT, SLP, lactation consultants[10,33,60,72,73]

Prevent	
Person/dyad factors	<ul><li>"Of utmost importance in decreasing symptoms of NAS is the opportunity for bonding and breastfeeding as mothers provide care for their newborns"[20(p404)]</li><li>"Active maternal participation is the best nonpharmacologic care,"[54(p e553)] to help mitigate withdrawal symptoms.</li><li>"Ideally, preparing the mother or primary caregiver to apply non-pharmacological techniques to help the newborn with NAS/NOWS and concurrently manage their own emotions should start prenatally."[19(p2)]</li><li>100% parental presence during hospitalization was associated with 8 fewer days of infant opioid therapy and lower mean Finnegan scores.[53]</li></ul>
Context (environmental) factors	
Task factors	<ul><li>Eat, Sleep, Console (ESC) approach to reduce need for pharmacologic treatment, shorten LOS, manage infant behaviors, build parent efficacy, and promote clustered care.[27,30,63,65,66,84]</li><li>Weight monitoring during ESC to avoid loss.[49]</li></ul>

(continued on next page)

Table 1
(continued)

EHP Intervention Approach	Target	Interventions
		• "Human breast milk (BM) is one non-pharmacologic measure that has been associated with decreased withdrawal symptoms and is indicated when mothers are stable,"[78(p877)] but not all mothers are able to breastfeed or provide expressed breast milk and support is needed.[11]
		• Using a multidisciplinary team considered best practice for parent education and support (nursing, nursing leadership, lactation, social work, child life, OT, SLP, physicians, trained volunteers)
		• Use of feeding specialists: OT, SLP, lactation consultants[10,33,60,72,73]
		• Recognition of potential challenges in the discharge location; infants with NAS/NOWS often inhabit stressful environments (eg, NICUs, chaotic homes or unstable housing, residential programs for mothers and children).[19]
		• Parent education regarding infant cues[10,11,19,28,66]
Create	Person/dyad factors	• Use strategies to optimize using non-pharmacologic measures before initiating pharmacologic management[30]
	Context (environmental) factors	• Ensure adequate lactation services[58]. NAS longer to achieve oral feeding; received fewer breastfeeding attempts
	Task factors	• Consider medical unit culture, for example, bottle-feeding vs breastfeeding,[37] non-pharm vs pharm,[49] and volume-driven vs infant-driven feeding goals
		• Provide trauma-informed and stigma-reducing care[12,26,49,85]
		• Create opportunities to address parent barriers (special formula costs, maternal nutrition, continued substance abuse, geographic location, education level, social support systems)
		• "Children born to mothers dependent on any substance are often exposed to other detrimental conditions including poverty, lack of resources and unstable home environments."[29(p2)]
		• Promote and use empowering parental messaging[30]
		• "Strategies aimed at integrally supporting opioid-exposed mothers and infants are vital for long-term clinical care, including an emphasis on prepregnancy, prenatal, and postnatal pain management; opioid use disorder treatment and recovery services; and neurocognitive, behavioral, and academic development through childhood and adolescence."[26(p173)]
		• Recognize non-pharmacologic interventions may need to vary based on geographic regions, demographics, and SES levels. Consider local social determinants.

Abbreviations: AR, added rice; IDDSI, International Dysphagia Diet Standardisation Initiative; NICUs, neonatal intensive care units; NNS, non-nutritive sucking; OT, occupational therapy; SLP, speech therapy.

Note: This table includes interventions that have been studied or are currently under study; critical appraisal is warranted based on strength of research design and methodology.

Alter interventions target contextual and/or task factors. Different than adapting or modifying the existing environment, altering interventions involves the health care professional trying to find the "best match" task or environment for the current skill level of the dyad, for example: moving an infant diagnosed with NAS/NOWS from a noisy location of the ICU to a quieter one; moving a nervous dyad to a room where one-to-one professional support is readily available/visible; shifting unit culture to a primary nursing model to encourage continuity of care and relationship-building; and altering care to include the ESC approach.

Adapt/Modify interventions can target environmental or task-related factors by changing or adjusting features to increase the infant–caregiver dyad's task (feeding) performance. Examples of adapt/modify at the environmental level include interventions targeting not only the physical environment around the baby (eg, darkening the room, decreasing the noise level) but also the social and cultural environments. Examples at the task level include interventions such as bottle changes, formula modifications, and schedule adaptations to support on-demand feeding.

Prevent interventions that can target person, environmental, or task-related factors and are implemented to "change the course of events when a negative outcome is predicted."[86(p627)] Interventions may include education on attachment, infant cues, developmental progression, aspiration, the sensory environment, and hospital policies.

Create interventions that can target person, environmental, or task-related factors. Interventions are "designed to promote and enrich performance" within a given context.[86(p627)] Both *Prevent* and *Create* interventions are implemented before a problem exists or if no problem exists.[51]

Taken together, the five intervention approaches allow critical care providers to use professional reasoning to consider the ecological influences present at each feeding (see **Table 1**). By attending to these myriad variables, professional caregivers can then generate numerous intervention options to build dyadic feeding success.

SUMMARY

Building on the work of Taylor and Maguire[22] and Velez and colleagues,[12,19] this review (1) reiterates the position that non-pharmacologic intervention should be considered in the management of withdrawal symptoms and support of the infant feeding dyad and (2) provides critical care providers with an updated picture of ecologically framed intervention strategies being used — or studied — to maximize feeding success in the NAS/NOWS population. Most of the evidence-based interventions featured in this review centered on Adapting or Modifying the contextual or task factors influencing feeding, followed by Establish/Restore interventions centered on person factors. Multiple Prevent interventions have been posited as contributors to feeding success, whereas fewer Create or Alter interventions have been examined in the literature. The challenge, therefore, is to consider the ecologic depth and breadth of non-pharmacologic interventions — especially those that extend beyond the bedside and reach to address the social determinants of health fueling the NAS/NOWS crisis.

The prevalence of NAS urges researchers and clinicians to develop effective strategies and techniques to treat and manage the poor feeding of infants exposed to substances in utero. Even with the clinical knowledge and experience that infants with NAS may be difficult to feed, there is limited research assessing techniques and schedules that are effective in managing successful feeding.[22]

In addition to the empirical study of infant feeding skills and behavior, the current imperative is to study how the infant–caregiver dyad's *transactional* feeding performance impacts feeding success. Beyond focused study of the dyad and bedside interventions, NAS/NOWS is considered a public health issue[44] which necessitates health care providers explore how environmental alterations and preventative or creative non-pharmacologic intervention could promote feeding success before any feeding challenges occur. Novel methods warrant future research; the safety and efficacy of non-pharmacologic interventions need further investigation to provide clear guidelines for clinical practice. Critical care providers are perfectly positioned to use advanced professional reasoning skills to comprehensively move through the seven steps of intervention planning proposed by Dunn[51] and doing so may ultimately empower the feeding dyad and promote feeding success at person, context, and task performance levels.

CLINICS CARE POINTS

- Neonatal abstinence syndrome or neonatal opioid withdrawal syndrome is known to disrupt feeding development and success.
- Non-pharmacologic interventions may be selected to mitigate withdrawal symptoms and may directly or indirectly influence feeding success.
- Interventions to address feeding challenges are shifting away from an infant-centric approach to one that focuses on the success of the infant–caregiver feeding dyad.
- The Ecology of Human Performance model[51] serves as a framework guiding professional reasoning for evidence-based intervention selection.
- More evidence is needed to further understand direct and indirect feeding interventions to support feeding dyad success.

DISCLOSURE

The author has no financial, commercial, or research-related competing interests to disclose.

REFERENCES

1. Filteau J, Coo H, Dow K. Trends in incidence of neonatal abstinence syndrome in Canada and associated healthcare resource utilization. Drug Alcohol Depend 2018;185:313–21.
2. Tolia V, Patrick S, Bennett M, et al. Increasing incidence of neonatal abstinence syndrome in US neonatal ICUs. Obstet Anesth Digest 2016;36(1):38. https://doi.org/10.1097/01.aoa.0000479516.96285.5d.
3. Zyoud SH, Al-Jabi SW, Shahwan MJ, et al. Global research production in neonatal abstinence syndrome: a bibliometric analysis. World J Clin Pediatr 2022;11(3):307–20.
4. CDC - Centers for Disease Control and Prevention. (n.d.) Available at: https://www.cdc.gov/pregnancy/opioids/data.html#:~:text=Neonatal%20Abstinence%20Syndrome&text=That%20is%20approximately%20one%20baby,59%20newborns%20diagnosed%20every%20day. Accessed September 3, 2023.
5. Patrick SW, Lorch SA. It is time to ACT NOW to improve quality for opioid-exposed infants. Pediatrics 2021;147(1). https://doi.org/10.1542/peds.2020-028340. e2020028340.

6. Hirai AH, Ko JY, Owens PL, et al. Neonatal abstinence syndrome and maternal opioid-related diagnoses in the U.S., 2010-2017. JAMA 2021;325(2):146–55.

7. Kozhimannil KB, Chantarat T, Ecklund AM, et al. Maternal opioid use disorder and Neonatal Abstinence Syndrome among rural US residents, 2007-2014. J Rural Health 2019;35(1):122–32.

8. Mensah NA, Madden EF, Qeadan F. Risk of feeding problems among infants with Neonatal Abstinence Syndrome: a retrospective cohort study. Adv Neonatal Care 2023;23(3):254–63.

9. Villapiano NL, Winkelman TN, Kozhimannil KB, et al. Rural and urban differences in Neonatal Abstinence Syndrome and maternal opioid use, 2004 to 2013. JAMA Pediatr 2017;171(2):194–6.

10. Anbalagan, S.D. & Mendez, M.D. Updated 2023 Jul 21. Neonatal Abstinence Syndrome. In: StatPearls Internet. Treasure Island (FL): StatPearls Publishing. https://www.ncbi.nlm.nih.gov/books/NBK551498/.

11. Pahl A, Pahl A, Young L, et al. Non-pharmacological care for opioid withdrawal in newborns. Cochrane Database Syst Rev 2020;12. https://doi.org/10.1002/14651858.cd013217.pub2.

12. Velez ML, Jordan C, Jansson LM. Reconceptualizing non-pharmacologic approaches to Neonatal Abstinence Syndrome (NAS) and Neonatal Opioid Withdrawal Syndrome (NOWS): a theoretical and evidence–based approach. Part II: the clinical application of nonpharmacologic care for NAS/NOWS. Neurotoxicol Teratol 2021b;88:107032.

13. Wachman EM, Farrer LA. The genetics and epigenetics of neonatal abstinence syndrome. Semin Fetal Neonatal Med 2019;24(2):105–10. https://doi.org/10.1016/j.siny.2019.01.002.

14. Yen E, Gaddis N, Jantzie L, et al. A review of the genomics of neonatal abstinence syndrome. Front Genet 2023;14. https://doi.org/10.3389/fgene.2023.1140400.

15. Jansson LM, Patrick SW. Neonatal abstinence syndrome. Pediatr Clin 2019;66(2):353–67.

16. McQueen K, Murphy-Oikonen J. Neonatal abstinence syndrome. N Engl J Med 2016;375:2468–79. https://doi.org/10.1056/NEJMra1600879.

17. Maguire DJ, Rowe MA, Spring H, et al. Patterns of disruptive feeding behaviors in infants with neonatal abstinence syndrome. Adv Neonatal Care 2015;15(6):429–39. https://doi.org/10.1097/anc.0000000000000204.

18. Maichuk GT, Zahorodny W, Marshall R. Use of positioning to reduce the severity of neonatal narcotic withdrawal syndrome. J Perinatol 1999;19(7):510–3.

19. Velez ML, Jordan C, Jansson LM. Reconceptualizing non-pharmacologic approaches to neonatal abstinence syndrome (NAS) and neonatal opioid withdrawal syndrome (NOWS): a theoretical and evidence-based approach. Neurotoxicol Teratol 2021a;88:107020.

20. McQueen K, Taylor C, Murphy-Oikonen J. A systematic review of newborn feeding method and outcomes related to Neonatal Abstinence Syndrome. J Obstet Gynecol Neonatal Nurs 2019;48(4):1–10. https://doi.org/10.1016/j.jogn.2019.03.004.

21. Righi L, Di Gloria A, Brussolo N, et al. Nursing interventions and assessment tool for neonatal abstinence syndrome (NAS): a case report. Journal of Pediatric and Neonatal Individualized Medicine 2023;12(2):e120209. https://doi.org/10.7363/120209.

22. Taylor K, Maguire D. A review of feeding practices in infants with neonatal abstinence syndrome. Adv Neonatal Care 2020;20(6):430–9.

23. Wu D, Carre C. The impact of breastfeeding on health outcomes for infants diagnosed with Neonatal Abstinence Syndrome: a review. Cureus 2018;10(7):e3061. https://doi.org/10.7759/cureus.3061.

24. Ghazanfarpour M, Najafi MN, Roozbeh N, et al. Therapeutic approaches for neonatal abstinence syndrome: a systematic review of randomized clinical trials. Daru: Journal of Faculty of Pharmacy 2019;27(1):423–31. Tehran University of Medical Sciences.

25. Zankl A, Martin J, Davey JG, et al. Opioid treatment for opioid withdrawal in newborn infants. Cochrane Database Syst Rev 2021;7(7):CD002059.

26. Jilani SM, Giroir BP. Neonatal Abstinence Syndrome: leveraging health information technology to develop a data-driven national policy approach. Publ Health Rep 2020;135(2):173–6.

27. Grossman MR, Berkwitt AK, Osborn RR, et al. An initiative to improve the quality of care of infants with neonatal abstinence syndrome. Pediatrics 2017;139(6): e20163360.

28. Holmes AV, Atwood EC, Whalen B, et al. Rooming-in to treat neonatal abstinence syndrome: improved family-centered care at a lower cost. Pediatrics 2016; 137(6):e20152929.

29. Mills-Huffnagle S, Nyland JE. Potential problems and solutions of opioid-based treatment in neonatal opioid withdrawal syndrome (NOWS): a scoping review protocol. BMJ Open 2023;13:e067883.

30. Ponder KL, Egesdal C, Kuller J, et al. Project Console: a quality improvement initiative for neonatal abstinence syndrome in a children's hospital level IV neonatal intensive care unit. BMJ Open Quality 2021;10:e001079. https://doi.org/10.1136/bmjoq-2020-001079.

31. Wachman EM, Schiff DM, Silverstein M. Neonatal abstinence syndrome: advances in diagnosis and treatment. JAMA 2018;319(13):1362–74.

32. Capilouto GJ, Cunningham TJ, Desai N. Quantifying the impact of common feeding interventions on nutritive sucking performance using a commercially available smart bottle. J Perinat Neonatal Nurs 2019;22(4):331–9.

33. Oostlander SA, Falla JA, Dow K, et al. Occupational therapy management strategies for infants with neonatal abstinence syndrome: a scoping review. Occup Ther Health Care 2019;33(2):197–226.

34. Mangat AK, Schmolzer GM, Kraft WK. Pharmacological and non-pharmacological treatments for neonatal abstinence syndrome (NAS). Semin Fetal Neonatal Med 2019;24:133–41.

35. MacMillan KDL, Rendon CP, Verma K, et al. Association of rooming-in with outcomes for Neonatal Abstinence Syndrome: a systematic review and meta-analysis. JAMA Pediatr 2018;172(4):345–51.

36. Jackson HJ, Lopez C, Miller S, et al. Feasibility of auricular acupressure as an adjunct treatment for neonatal opioid withdrawal syndrome (NOWS). Subst Abuse 2021;42(3):348–57. https://journals.sagepub.com/doi/10.1080/08897077.2020.1784360.

37. Cardin AD, Conner P, Hedrick HR, et al. Understanding feeding complexity and culture in the NICU: a qualitative study. J Neonatal Nurs 2023;1–8. https://doi.org/10.1016/j.jnn.2023.04.002.

38. Als H. A synactive model of neonatal behavioral organization: framework for the assessment of neurobehavioral development in the premature infant and for support of infants and parents in the neonatal intensive care environment. Phys Occup Ther Pediatr 1986;6. https://doi.org/10.1080/j006v06n03_02.

39. Rhooms L, Dow K, Brandon C, et al. Effect of unimodal and multimodal sensori-motor interventions on oral feeding outcomes in preterm infants. Adv Neonatal Care 2019;19(1):E3–20. https://doi.org/10.1097/anc.0000000000000546.

40. Bertoncelli N, Cuomo G, Cattani S, et al. Oral feeding competences of healthy preterm infants: a review. Int J Pediatr 2012;2012:896257.

41. Bowman OJ, Hagan JL, Toruno RM, Wiggin MM. Identifying Aspiration Among Infants in Neonatal Intensive Care Units Through Occupational Therapy Feeding Evaluations. Am J Occup Ther 2020;74(1):7401205080p1–7401205080p9.

42. Tamilia E, Taffoni F, Formica D, et al. Technological solutions and main indices for the assessment of newborns' nutritive sucking: a review. Sensors (Basel) 2014; 14(1):634–58.

43. Hart BJ, Viswanathan S, Jadcherla SR. Persistent feeding difficulties among infants with fetal opioid exposure: mechanisms and clinical reasoning. J Matern Fetal Neonatal Med 2019;32(21):3633–9.

44. Yen E, Maron JL. Aberrant feeding and growth in neonates with prenatal opioid exposure: evidence of neuromodulation and behavioral changes. Frontiers in Pediatrics 2022;9:1–8.

45. Griffith TT, Bell AF, Vincent C, et al. Oral feeding success: a concept analysis. Adv Neonatal Care 2018;19(1):21–31.

46. Lau C, Smith EO. A novel approach to assess oral feeding skills of preterm infants. Neonatology 2011;100(1):64–70.

47. LaGasse LL, Messinger D, Lester BM, et al. Prenatal drug exposure and maternal and infant feeding behavior. Arch Dis Child Fetal Neonatal 2003;88:F391–9.

48. McGlothen-Bell K, Cleveland L, Recto P, et al. Feeding behaviors in infants with prenatal opioid exposure: an integrative review. Adv Neonatal Care 2020;20(5): 374–83.

49. Perez C. *Exploring Infant Massage as Standard Nonpharmacological Treatment for Neonatal Opioid Withdrawal Syndrome*. Doctoral dissertation, Walden University; 2022. p. 1–232.

50. Dunn W, Brown C, McGuigan A. The ecology of human performance: a framework for considering the effect of context. Am J Occup Ther 1994;48(7):595–607.

51. Dunn W. The ecological model of occupation. In: Hinojosa J, Kramer P, Brasic Royeen C, editors. Perspectives on human occupation – theories underlying practice. 2nd edition. Davis: F.A; 2017. p. 207–35.

52. Pados B, Fuller K. Establishing a foundation for optimal feeding outcomes in the NICU. Nursing for Women's Health 2020;24(3):202–9.

53. Howard MB, Schiff DM, Penwill N, et al. Impact of parental presence at infants' bedside on Neonatal Abstinence Syndrome. Hosp Pediatr 2017;7(2):63–9.

54. Kocherlakota. Neonatal abstinence syndrome. Pediatrics 2014;134(2):e547–61. https://doi.org/10.1542/peds.2013-3524.

55. Williams LR, Gebler-Wolfe M, Grisham LM, et al. "Babywearing" in the NICU: an intervention for infants with neonatal abstinence syndrome. Adv Neonatal Care 2020;20(6):440–9. https://doi.org/10.1097/ANC.0000000000000788.

56. Lembeck AL, Tuttle D, Locke R, et al. Breastfeeding and formula selection in neonatal abstinence syndrome. Am J Perinatol 2021;38:1488–93. https://doi.org/10.1055/s-0040-1713754.

57. Liu A, Juarez J, Nair A, et al. Feeding modalities and the onset of the neonatal abstinence syndrome. Frontiers in Pediatrics 2015;3:14. https://www.frontiersin.org/articles/10.3389/fped.2015.00014/full.

58. Nagy S, Dow K, Fucile S. Oral feeding outcomes in infants born with neonatal abstinence syndrome. J Perinat Neonatal Nurs 2023. https://doi.org/10.1097/JPN.0000000000000741.

59. Newman AI, Mauer-Vakil D, Coo H, et al. Rooming-in for infants at risk for neonatal abstinence syndrome: outcomes 5 years following its introduction as the standard of care at one hospital. Am J Perinatol 2022;39(8):897–903.

60. Pritham UA. Breastfeeding promotion for management of neonatal abstinence syndrome. J Obstet Gynecol Neonatal Nurs 2013;42(5):517–26.

61. Rinaldi K, Maguire D. Verbal behavior of mothers with opioid use disorder while feeding infants with neonatal opioid withdrawal syndrome. Adv Neonatal Care 2023;23(4):e96–105.

62. Welle-Strand GK, Skurtveit S, Jansson LM, et al. Breastfeeding reduces the need for withdrawal treatment in opioid-exposed infants. ActaPaediatrica 2013;102(11):1060–6.

63. Young LW, Ounpraseuth ST, Merhar SL, et al. Eat, Sleep, Console Approach or usual care for neonatal opioid withdrawal. N Engl J Med 2023;388l:2326–37.

64. Radziewicz RA, Wright-Esber S, Zupancic J, et al. Safety of reiki therapy for newborns at risk for neonatal abstinence syndrome. Holist Nurs Pract 2018;32(2):63–70. https://doi.org/10.1097/HNP.0000000000000251.

65. Blount T, Painter A, Freeman E, et al. Reduction in length of stay and morphine use for NAS with the "Eat, Sleep, Console" method. Hosp Pediatr 2019;9(8):615–23.

66. Wachman EM, Houghton M, Melvin P, et al. A quality improvement initiative to implement the eat, sleep, console neonatal opioid withdrawal syndrome care tool in Massachusetts' PNQIN collaborative. J Perinatol 2020;40(10):1560–9.

67. Jackson HJ, López C, Miller S, et al. Neonatal abstinence syndrome: an integrative review of neonatal acupuncture to inform a protocol for adjunctive treatment. Adv Neonatal Care 2019;19(3):165–78.

68. Jansson LM, Patrick SW. Neonatal Abstinence Syndrome. Pediatr Clin North Am 2019;66(2):353–67.

69. Urlesberger B, Cabano R, Soll G, et al. Acupuncture for neonatal abstinence syndrome in newborn infants (Protocol). Cochrane Database Syst Rev 2023;8:CD014160. https://doi.org/10.1002/14651858.CD014160.

70. Rana D, Garde K, Elabiad MT, et al. Whole body massage for newborns: a report on non-invasive methodology for neonatal opioid withdrawal syndrome. J Neonatal Perinat Med 2022;15(3):559–65.

71. Hudak ML, Tan RC, committee on drugs, committee on fetus and newborn, & American Academy of Pediatrics. Neonatal drug withdrawal. Pediatrics 2012;129(2):e540–60.

72. Schaaf RC, Dumont RL, Arbesman M, et al. Efficacy of occupational therapy using Ayres Sensory Integration®: a systematic review. Am J Occup Ther 2018;72(1). 7201190010p1.

73. Proctor-Williams K, 1 Nov. The opioid crisis on our caseloads. ASHA Leader 2018.

74. Bloch-Salisbury E, Bogen D, Vining M, et al. Study design and rationale for a randomized controlled trial to assess effectiveness of stochastic vibrotactile mattress stimulation versus standard non-oscillating crib mattress for treating hospitalized opioid-exposed newborns. Contemporary Clinical Trials Communications 2021;21. https://doi.org/10.1016/j.conctc.2021.100737.

75. D'Apolito K. Comparison of a rocking bed and standard bed for decreasing withdrawal symptoms in drug-exposed infants. American Journal of Maternal/Child Nursing 1999;24(3):138–44.

76. Zuzarte I, Indic P, Barton B, et al. stimulation, Vibrotactile stimulation: a non-pharmacological intervention for opioid-exposed newborns. PLoS One 2017; 12(4):e0175981. https://doi.org/10.1371/journal.pone.0175981.
77. Pandey R, Kanike N, Ibrahim M, et al. Lactose-free infant formula does not change outcomes of neonatal abstinence syndrome (NAS): a randomized clinical trial. J Perinatol 2021;41(3):598–605.
78. Favara MT, Carola D, Jensen E, et al. Maternal breast milk feeding and length of treatment in infants with neonatal abstinence syndrome. J Perinatol 2019;39(6): 876–82.
79. Pados BF, Feaster V. Effect of formula type and preparation on International Dysphagia Diet Standardisation Initiative Thickness Level and milk flow rates from bottle teats. Am J Speech Lang Pathol 2021;30(1):260–5.
80. Kurup U, Merchant N. Neonatal abstinence syndrome: management and current concepts. Paediatr Child Health 2020;31(1):24–31.
81. Bell N, Harding C. An investigation of the flow rates of disposable bottle teats used to feed preterm and medically fragile infants in neonatal units across the UK in comparison with flow rates of commercially available bottle teats. Speech Lang Hear 2019;22(3):1–9.
82. Pados BF, Park J, Dodrill P. Know the flow: milk flow rates from bottle nipples used in the hospital and after discharge. Adv Neonatal Care 2019;19(1):32–41.
83. Daniel JM, Davidson LN, Havens JR, et al. Aromatherapy as an adjunctive therapy for neonatal abstinence syndrome: a pilot study. Journal of Opioid Management 2020;16(2):119–25.
84. Casavant SG, Fleming M, Hussain N, et al. Integrative review of the assessment of newborns with neonatal abstinence syndrome. Journal of Obstetrical Gynecological Neonatal Nursing 2021;50(5):539–48.
85. Klukken A, Wasmuth S. Applying the Ecological Model of Human Performance and the SlutWalk Movement to support those affected by rape culture in the context of occupational therapy. Open Journal of Occupational Therapy 2023; 11(3):1–5.
86. Brown C. Ecological model of health performance. In: Boyt Schell BA, Gillen G, editors. *Willard and Spackman's occupational therapy.* 13th edition. the Netherlands: Wolters Kluwer; 2019. p. 622–32.

Breastfeeding Practice Before Bottle-Feeding

An Initiative to Increase the Rate of Breastfeeding for Preterm Infants at the Time of Neonatal Intensive Care Unit Discharge

Raylene Phillips, MD, MA, IBCLC[a,b,c],*,
Dawn VanNatta, OTR/L, SWC, CNT, CLEC[c,1],
Jenny Chu, MA, OTR/L, SWC, IBCLC[c,1], Allison Best, DNP, FNP, RN, BSN[c,1],
Pamela Ruiz, RN, BS, IBCLC[c,1], Tonya Oswalt, RN, BSN, IBCLC[c,1],
Dianne Wooldridge, RN, IBCLC[c,1], Elba Fayard, MD[a,b,c,1]

KEYWORDS

- Breastfeeding • Bottle-feeding • Oral feeding • Preterm infant • NICU discharge

KEY POINTS

- We are introducing direct breastfeeding practice for preterm infants before bottle-feeding, which is associated with increased breastfeeding rates and breast milk feeding at the time of neonatal intensive care unit (NICU) discharge.
- Preterm infants may learn to breastfeed more easily if allowed to practice breastfeeding before introducing bottles.
- Preterm babies and their mothers who are highly motivated to breastfeed can be supported in direct breastfeeding without increasing the time to full oral feeds or length of NICU stay.

INTRODUCTION

The benefits of breast milk for babies and their mothers have been well documented for many years.[1–3] In the United States, more than 80% of mothers want to breastfeed

[a] Loma Linda University Children's Hospital, Neonatology Division, 11175 Campus Street, CP 11121, Loma Linda, CA 92350, USA; [b] Loma Linda University School of Medicine, Department of Pediatrics, Division of Neonatology, 11175 Campus Street, Loma Linda, CA 92350, USA; [c] Loma Linda University Children's Hospital, Unit 3700, 11234 Anderson Street, Loma Linda, CA, 92354, USA
[1] Co-author
* Corresponding author. Loma Linda University Children's Hospital, Neonatology Division, 11175 Campus Street, CP 11121, Loma Linda, CA 92350, USA.
E-mail address: rphillips@llu.edu

Crit Care Nurs Clin N Am 36 (2024) 251–260
https://doi.org/10.1016/j.cnc.2023.12.005
0899-5885/24/© 2024 Elsevier Inc. All rights reserved.

their babies enough to initiate breastfeeding.[4] For many mothers, their desire to breastfeed does not change just because their babies are born prematurely.[5] Our 84-bed Level 4 neonatal intensive care unit (NICU), like other NICUs worldwide, has tried for several years to better support NICU mothers who wish to breastfeed their premature or sick infants.

More than 60% of mothers who plan to breastfeed do not breastfeed as long as they had intended.[6] Having a preterm infant in the NICU is just one of many reasons mothers may not reach their breastfeeding goals. There are many known barriers to breastfeeding in the NICU, including the challenge of establishing and maintaining a sufficient milk supply.[7] Although our NICU had succeeded in better supporting mothers in pumping breast milk, and our rates of breast milk feeding at the time of NICU discharge had increased, our rates of direct breastfeeding remained low. Many babies were going home from the NICU without ever having breastfed directly at their mother's breast.

One of the barriers to breastfeeding in the NICU is the reality that many mothers cannot be present in the NICU at feeding times. Some live a long distance from the NICU. Many have other children at home and/or transportation challenges.

Another unintended barrier is that NICU nurses are very skilled at bottle-feeding preterm infants, and many mothers think that their babies will get home faster if they just let the experts feed their babies. Some nurses and even physicians support this belief by telling mothers that learning to breastfeed will delay the achievement of full oral feedings and NICU discharge. Mothers are often encouraged by well-meaning, but misinformed, staff to focus on bottle-feeding so their babies can get to full oral feedings sooner. Many are told their baby can learn to breastfeed at home. However, this is not how it works for successful breastfeeding to occur. Experience has shown that many babies will refuse to breastfeed if they become accustomed to bottle-feeding first. However, if they learn to breastfeed first, most babies will be willing to go back and forth between breast and bottle-feeding.

Avoiding bottles by using nasal gastric tube supplements to breastfeeding instead of bottle-feeding supplements while transitioning to oral feeds has been shown to increase breastfeeding rates at the time of NICU discharge without increasing NICU hospitalization.[8–10] One study found increased breastfeeding rates at the time of NICU discharge and increased breastfeeding rates at 3 days, 3 months, and 6 months after discharge home.[10] A 2021 Cochrane Review evaluated 7 trials (5 used a cup-feeding strategy, 1 used tube feeding, and 1 used a novel teat) involving 1152 preterm infants to identify the effects of avoidance of bottle-feeds during the establishment of breastfeeding on the likelihood of successful breastfeeding and concluded that avoiding the use of bottles when preterm infants need supplementary feeds probably increases the extent of any breastfeeding at discharge, and may improve any and exclusive breastfeeding up to 6 months after discharge.[11]

In a study to determine factors associated with successful direct breastfeeding of preterm infants, Casey and colleagues found that having the first oral feeding attempt at the breast was a critical predictor of breastfeeding success at the time of hospital discharge.[12] More days between the first breastfeeding and the introduction of a bottle have been associated with a higher chance of breastfeeding at the time of NICU discharge.[13]

It did not seem feasible to avoid all bottle-feeding in our NICU, so we developed a protocol to support mothers who wished to breastfeed their preterm babies in the NICU by introducing breastfeeding practice first before bottle-feeding and then supporting both breastfeeding and bottle-feeding while transitioning from gavage tube feedings to full oral feedings. We tested its effectiveness through a quality improvement (QI) initiative.

METHODS

A QI study was created by a multidisciplinary team (NICU physicians, lactation consultants, occupational therapists, and nurses) with the primary aim to increase the rate of preterm infants who were breastfeeding at the time of NICU discharge. A secondary aim was to determine if focusing on breastfeeding before bottle-feeding would influence the time to full oral feedings or the length of hospital stay. This study was deemed to be quality improvement and thus exempt from Institutional Review Board (IRB) approval. This article was developed using guidelines from the Revised Standards for Quality Improvement Reporting Excellence.[14]

A preterm breastfeeding pathway (PBP) was created with our primary aim in mind. The target population for this pathway is mothers who desire to breastfeed their preterm babies in the NICU and have an adequate milk supply (verified by the NICU lactation consultant) and whose preterm baby is on full gavage feeds and is ready to begin oral feedings (confirmed by the neonatologist and the NICU feeding specialists).

NICU feeding specialists in our NICU include International Board-Certified Lactation Consultants and occupational therapists. Lactation consultants meet with all NICU mothers within 24 hours of their baby's admission to determine their feeding goals, give verbal and written education about the many important benefits of mother's own milk for preterm babies, and support early and regular breastmilk expression with an electric pump. Occupational therapists meet with mothers of preterm infants to discuss the importance of positive oral experiences with pacifiers and the mother's nipple during skin-to-skin contact whenever the baby is interested—even before readiness for oral feeding. Mothers who desire to breastfeed are introduced to the PBP and asked if they would like to participate.

Each mother's availability to be in the NICU for breastfeeding practice is determined, and it is explained that if she can be in the NICU for at least 3 feedings a day for the first 72 hours of oral feeds, this will give her baby the opportunity to practice breastfeeding first before bottle-feeding is introduced, which may improve the chances of successful breastfeeding by the time the baby is ready for NICU discharge. Every effort is made to have these conversations in a compassionate, nonjudgmental manner, assuring mothers who cannot be in the NICU as often as they wish that their babies will be well cared for in their absence and that they will be welcomed and supported in breastfeeding whenever they can be present when their baby is ready for oral feedings.

A primary goal of the PBP is to prioritize first oral feeding at the breast for all pumping mothers. Mothers who have been pumping for weeks or months deserve to give their babies their first oral feeding at the breast, even if the baby transfers very little milk at first. When a baby is ready for oral feedings, the mother is notified, and arrangements are made for her to be present for the first oral feeding at the breast. The first time breastfeeding is a significant milestone for all mothers who desire to breastfeed, but it is especially important to mothers of preterm infants, and it should be marked with appropriate acknowledgements and celebrations. If a mother cannot get to the NICU in a reasonable length of time (within a day or two), then oral feeding is not delayed, and bottle-feeding practice is begun with breastfeeding support whenever the mother can be present.

For mothers who can be present in the NICU for the first 72 hours of oral feeds, the PBP has 2 stages: (1) during the first 72 hours and (2) after the first 72 hours. During the first 72 hours after the baby's first oral feeding, whenever a mother is present, cue-based breastfeeding practice is supported with the administration of full gavage feedings, and bottle-feeding practice is deferred. After 72 hours of breastfeeding practice, babies continue to practice cue-based breastfeeding with full gavage support when the mother is present and practice cue-based bottle-feeding with gavage support when the mother is absent.

If a mother cannot be present for at least 3 feedings a day, we still make every effort for the baby to have the first oral feeding at the breast and support cue-based breastfeeding practice whenever the mother is present but whenever the mother is absent, the baby is offered cue-based bottle-feeding practice with gavage support. Bottle-feeding practice is not deferred if a mother cannot be present for at least 3 sessions of breastfeeding practice during the first 72 hours of oral feedings. An algorithm was created to help guide nurses caring for babies whose mothers desire to breastfeed (**Fig. 1**, **Box 1**).

Infant-led, cue-based feeding principles are used for all feeding attempts. A preterm infant feeding readiness scale[15] is used to determine if baby is demonstrating appropriate feeding cues. Until babies are 35 weeks of corrected gestational age (CGA), the entire feeding is given via a gavage feeding tube while the baby practices breastfeeding. Preterm babies less than 35 weeks CGA are not expected to take much volume, so no effort is made to estimate intake. If a baby seems to be breastfeeding better than expected, the NICU lactation consultant or occupational therapists (who also have breastfeeding training) are consulted to consider readiness for estimating breastfeeding intake.

When babies are practicing breastfeeding, nurses are encouraged to avoid offering a bottle to finish a feeding after breastfeeding. If, after a pause, the baby is still showing

Preterm Breastfeeding Pathway

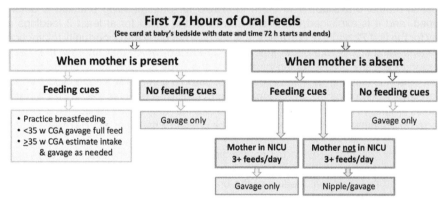

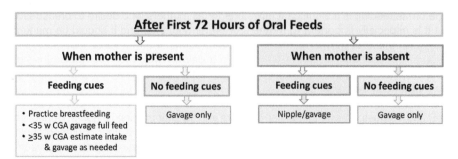

Fig. 1. PBP algorithm.

Box 1
Summary of preterm breastfeeding pathway algorithm

- During the first 72 hours of oral feeds, if mother *can* be present for at least 3 feeds a day:
  - When mother is present, baby gets breastfeeding practice with gavage support
  - When mother is absent, baby gets gavage feeds only with no bottles
- During the first 72 hours of oral feeds, if mother *cannot* be present for at least 3 feeds a day:
  - When mother is present, baby gets breastfeeding practice with gavage support
  - When mother is absent, baby gets bottle-feeding practice with gavage support
- After the first 72 hours, all babies practice breastfeeding when mother is present and practice bottle-feeding when mother is absent

All oral feedings are infant-led and cue-based feeds.

---

feeding cues, babies are supported in continuing to breastfeed. If the baby stops showing feeding cues during a breastfeeding, gavage tube feeding is used to finish the feeding rather than a bottle (to be consistent with our cue-based feeding practice).

Two methods are available to estimate breastfeeding intake: (1) pre–breastfeeding and post–breastfeeding weights using a breastfeeding baby-weight scale designed for this purpose (**Box 2**), or (2) quality and duration of latch and suckling as determined by the mother and nurse together (**Box 3**). The breastfeeding baby-weight scale available in our NICU is the Medela Babyweigh Scale (Medela; Baar, Switzerland). Nurses are encouraged to involve mothers in choosing and actively participating in the method most appropriate for their baby. Nurses document estimated breastfeeding intake in the hospital's electronic medical record and indicate the method used to determine the estimated volume. Gavage tube feeding volumes are adjusted until the baby is weaned off gavage feedings.

We evaluated outcomes for 3 groups of preterm babies born at less than 33 weeks gestational age (GA) based on how they were fed during the first 72 hours of oral feedings. Qualification criteria for mothers included a desire to breastfeed and adequate milk supply from pumping (verified with the NICU lactation consultant). Qualification criteria for their babies included tolerating full gavage feeding and readiness to begin oral feedings (confirmed with the neonatologist and the NICU occupational therapist). We documented birth gestational age, birth weight, and gender. Outcomes measured included the following:

Box 2
Preterm breastfeeding pathway: calculating estimated breastfeeding intake using a breastfeeding baby-weight scale

Calculating Estimated Breastfeeding Intake

Medela Babyweigh Scale
  Babies ≥35 wk CGA
- Use for babies with no IV or respiratory support headgear
- Weigh baby before and after breastfeeding per scale directions
  - Mothers can learn this skill and can often do it independently
- Calculate estimated milk intake (1 g = 1 mL) and gavage remainder of feed
- Document breastfeeding intake in "Estimated Breastfeeding Amount (mL)"
- Document "*by scale/pathway*" in Comments section
- Document "Breastfeeding count" and "Amount of Time Breastfeeding"
- Document gavage volume in "Breast Milk-tube"

Box 3
Preterm breastfeeding pathway: calculating estimated breastfeeding intake using quality and duration of latch and suckling

Calculating Estimated Breastfeeding Intake

Quality and duration of latch and suckling
  Babies ≥35 weeks CGA
  • Involve mothers in evaluation of latch and suckling
  • Poor latch and/or weak suck - > gavage full feeding
  • Good latch and strong suck
    ○ Less than 5 min -> gavage full feeding
    ○ 5–10 min - > gavage 3/4 feeding
    ○ 11–15 min - > gavage 1/2 feeding
    ○ 16–20 min - > gavage 1/4 feeding
    ○ Greater than 20 min - > no gavage
  • Document breastfeeding intake in "estimated breastfeeding amount (mL)"
  • Document *"by Latch/pathway"* in Comments section
  • Document "breastfeeding count" and "amount of time breastfeeding"
  • Document gavage volume in "breast milk-tube"

• Breastfeeding, breast milk feeding (with bottle), or formula feeding at NICU discharge
• CGA at first and full oral feeds
• Time (days) from first to full oral feeds
• CGA and day of life at NICU discharge

RESULTS

Seventy-five preterm infants born at less than 33 weeks GA who had met the criteria for the PBP were discharged from our NICU between April and December 2019. By chart review, we compared 3 groups of babies based on how they were fed during the first 72 hours of oral feedings, including (1) babies who received 72 hours of breast-feeding practice before introducing a bottle (breast only, n-27), (2) babies who were introduced to bottle-feeding with or before breastfeeding (bottle/breast, n = 15), and (3) babies who were primarily bottle-fed (bottle only, n = 33).

Babies who received 72 hours of breastfeeding practice before being introduced to a bottle (breast only) compared with babies who received bottle-feeding with or before breastfeeding practice (bottle/breast) or babies who were primarily bottle-fed (bottle only) during the first 72 hours of oral feeding had significantly higher rates of both breastfeeding (88.9%, 66.7%, and 3%, respectively, $P < .001$) and breast milk feeding (100%, 86.7%, and 39.4%, respectively, $P<.001$) at time of NICU discharge. There were no statistical differences between groups in birth GA, birth weight, or gender, CGA at first or full oral feeds, time (days) from first to full oral feeds, or in days of life or CGA at time of NICU discharge (**Table 1**).

DISCUSSION

We found that supporting mothers who wished to breastfeed their preterm infants in the NICU by making every effort to have the baby's first oral feeding at the breast and by delaying the introduction of bottle-feeding for 72 hours was successful in increasing the rate of direct breastfeeding at the time of NICU discharge. This strategy did not stand alone and included our long-standing support of NICU mothers beginning as soon as possible after birth. NICU lactation consultants visit mothers in their

Table 1			
Outcomes for 3 groups of preterm babies based on how they were fed during the first 72 h of oral feeding			
Groups: first 72 h of oral feeding			
Breast Only	Bottle/Breast	Bottle Only	
n = 27	n = 15	n = 33	
Percent breastfeeding at NICU discharge			
89%	67%	3%	P<.001
Percent with breast milk feeds at NICU discharge			
100%	87%	39%	P<.001
Time to reach full oral feeds (days)			
22.1 ± 9.8	19.7 ± 9.6	22.4 ± 13.3	P = .593
CGA at full oral feeds (weeks)			
36 (34–40)	37 (34–43)	36 (34–45)	P = .408
Days of life at NICU discharge			
50.7 ± 26.6	65.9 ± 18.7	60.2 ± 24.5	P = .126
CGA at NICU discharge (weeks)			
37 (35–42)	38 (36–45)	37 (34–46)	P = .408

postpartum rooms to ensure they have a hospital electric pump, the correct-sized flange, and know how to use the pump. They are also taught how to store their milk and to understand that breast milk is "medicine" for their preterm infants. NICU lactation consultants continue to support pumping mothers throughout their baby's hospital stay. Early, frequent, and prolonged skin-to-skin contact is encouraged and facilitated. These long-standing support measures, however, had not resulted in increased rates of direct breastfeeding, which motivated us to find new ways to support mothers who wished to breastfeed their preterm infants in the NICU.

Supporting mothers in establishing and maintaining adequate breast milk volumes for their NICU babies is a priority in most NICUs. Still, support for direct breastfeeding presents unique challenges, including the need for the mother's presence and a requirement for more staff time and skill. It is easier to support mothers at a distance in pumping breast milk than to support them directly in positioning, latching, and pacing a preterm baby at the breast.

Multiple studies have demonstrated how vital breastfeeding is to many NICU mothers. While exploring the experience of preterm infants' mothers with milk expression and breastfeeding, Ikonen and colleagues found that despite the challenges of providing milk and the difficulties of breastfeeding in the NICU, mothers found breastfeeding helped to rebuild the interrupted connection with their babies; even learning how to express breast milk was an essential factor in connecting them with their preterm babies.[16]

Although direct breastfeeding at the time of NICU discharge is a worthy goal, a more important long-term goal is continued breastfeeding long after NICU discharge. All organizations that support breastfeeding recommend exclusive breastfeeding for the first 6 months and continued breastfeeding for 1 to 2 years after or as long as the mother and baby desire.[4]

Mothers of preterm infants often receive mixed messages about breastfeeding in the NICU, with a higher focus on pumping breast milk and early discharge than on breastfeeding. With adequate experience in direct breastfeeding, mothers can gain the knowledge and skills for successful breastfeeding at home.[17] Successful breastfeeding can be an empowering experience for mothers of preterm infants, whereas unsuccessful breastfeeding can induce feelings of disappointment and failure.[17]

Breastfeeding duration during the first year after birth for preterm infants has been associated with mothers' breastfeeding satisfaction.[18] Breastfeeding knowledge and self-efficacy are associated with breastfeeding duration at 6 months after discharge of preterm infants.[19] Achieving success in breastfeeding requires support for most mothers. Even if their babies are healthy and full-term, many mothers need assistance from someone more experienced or trained in breastfeeding in the first few days after birth. Helping mothers with preterm infants achieve breastfeeding success requires early and skilled breastfeeding support in the NICU so that mothers can gain the knowledge and experience to attain breastfeeding self-efficacy and develop trust in themselves and in their infant's ability to breastfeed.

NICU nurses play a critical role in helping mothers to breastfeed their preterm infants, and many studies around the world have shown ways they and other NICU professionals can provide consistent, evidence-based information to support mothers of preterm infants in expressing milk, skin-to-skin contact (kangaroo care), and breastfeeding in the NICU and at home after NICU discharge.[12–25]

A key feature of our QI study was making it possible for mothers who wished to breastfeed their preterm infants to have the experience of direct breastfeeding well before NICU discharge. In a study of 81 infants who were born at *less than* 32 weeks gestation, it was found that the earlier skin-to-skin contact (kangaroo care) was started, and the earlier parents were involved in feeding their preterm infants, the lower postmenstrual age they were at full oral feeds.[26] During skin-to-skin contact, preterm babies can become familiar with the mother's breast and nipple as preparation for breastfeeding when they are ready for oral feedings.

A small qualitative study of 9 mothers who had given birth to extremely preterm infants found themes that likely reflect those of many mothers of preterm babies. Despite their struggles with breast milk expression and difficulties with breastfeeding practice, these mothers had a strong will to provide breast milk for their infants. Their unifying request was for more support in order to be successful.[27] It is our responsibility as NICU professionals to provide that support to the mothers who desire it.

SUMMARY AND IMPLICATIONS

Preterm infants can be supported in learning to breastfeed successfully before leaving the NICU without increasing the time to full oral feeds or the length of NICU stay. If preterm infants get 3 days of focused direct breastfeeding practice before introducing a bottle, they are significantly more likely to be breastfeeding at the time of NICU discharge than if bottles were introduced first.

Although not all mothers can be present for a period of focused breastfeeding practice, we can support the subset of mothers who can be present at feeding times and are highly motivated to do so by their desire to breastfeed. This QI initiative demonstrated that by supporting these mothers and their preterm babies, we could achieve significantly increased breastfeeding and breast milk feeding rates at the time of NICU discharge.

LIMITATIONS

This was a small QI study conducted in a large Level 4 NICU in the Southwest United States. A larger research trial is needed to validate these QI study results.

CLINICS CARE POINTS

- Supporting direct breastfeeding practice before bottling feeding in the first 72 hours of oral feeding significantly increased the rates of direct breastfeeding and breast milk feedings (with bottle) at the time of NICU discharge for preterm infants born at less than 33 weeks GA.

- Supporting breastfeeding practice for preterm infants before introducing bottle-feeding did not increase the time to full oral feeds and did not delay the time of NICU discharge.

- Mothers who are highly motivated to breastfeed their preterm infants can be supported in doing so before NICU discharge without concerns about lengthening their baby's NICU hospitalization.

ACKNOWLEDGMENTS

The authors wish to express our gratitude to the mothers and babies who participated in this initiative and to all the NICU staff who supported it.

DISCLOSURE

None of the authors has commercial or financial conflicts of interest or funding sources.

REFERENCES

1. Gavine A, Shinwell SC, Buchanan P, et al. Support for healthy breastfeeding mothers with healthy term babies. Cochrane Database Syst Rev 2022;(10):CD001141.
2. Dieterich CM, Felice JP, O'Sullivan E, et al. Breastfeeding and health outcomes for the mother-infant dyad. Pediatr Clin North Am 2013;60(1):31–48.
3. Horta BL. Breastfeeding: Investing in the Future. Breastfeed Med 2019;14(S1): S11–2.
4. Center for Disease Control and Prevention. CDC 24/7: Saving Lives, Protecting People. Available at: https://www.cdc.gov/breastfeeding/data/facts.html. Accessed November 26, 2023.
5. Sweet L. Birth of a very low birth weight preterm infant and the intention to breastfeed 'naturally'. Women Birth 2008;21(1):13–20.
6. Odom EC, Li R, Scanlon KS, et al. Reasons for earlier than desired cessation of breastfeeding. Pediatrics 2013;131(3):e726–32.
7. Bujold M, Feeley N, Axelin A, et al. Expressing Human milk in the NICU: Coping Mechanisms and challenges Shape the Complex experience of Closeness and Separation. Adv Neonatal Care 2018;18(1):38–48.
8. Stine MJ. Breastfeeding the premature infant: a protocol without bottles. J Hum Lactation 1990;6:167–70.
9. Nye C. Transitioning premature infants from gavage to breast. Neonatal Netw 2008;27(1):7–13.
10. Kliethermes PA, Cross ML, Lanese MG, et al. Transitioning preterm infants with Nasogastric tube Supplementation: increased likelihood of breastfeeding. J Obstet Gynecol Neonatal Nurs 1999;28(3):264–73.
11. Allen E, Rumbold AR, Keir A, et al. Avoidance of bottles during the establishment of breastfeeds in preterm infants. Cochrane Database Syst Rev 2021;10(10): CD005252.

12. Casey L, Fucile S, Dow KE. Determinants of successful direct breastfeeding at hospital discharge in High-Risk premature infants. Breastfeed Med 2018;13(5): 346–51.

13. Briere CE, McGrath JM, Cong X, et al. Direct-breastfeeding premature infants in the neonatal intensive care Unit. J Hum Lact 2015;31(3):386–92.

14. Ogrinc G, Davies L, Goodman D, et al. SQUIRE 2.0 (Standards for quality improvement Reporting Excellence): Revised Publication guidelines from a Detailed Consensus Process. J Nurs Care Qual 2016;31(1):1–8.

15. Ludwig SM, Waitzman KA. Changing feeding documentation to reflect infant-driven feeding practice. Nborn Infant Nurs Rev 2007;7:155–60.

16. Ikonen R, Paavilainen E, Kaunonen M. Preterm infants' mothers' experiences with milk expression and breastfeeding: an integrative review. Adv Neonatal Care 2015;15(6):394–406.

17. Niela-Vilén H, Axelin A, Melender HL, et al. Aiming to be a breastfeeding mother in a neonatal intensive care unit and at home: a thematic analysis of peer-support group discussion in social media. Matern Child Nutr 2015;11(4):712–26.

18. Ericson J, Lampa E, Flacking R. Breastfeeding satisfaction post hospital discharge and associated factors — a longitudinal cohort study of mothers of preterm infants. Int Breastfeed J 2021;16(1):28.

19. Jiang X, Jiang H. Factors associated with post NICU discharge exclusive breast-feeding rate and duration amongst first-time mothers of preterm infants in Shanghai: a longitudinal cohort study. Int Breastfeed J 2022;17(1):34.

20. Isaacson LJ. Steps to successfully breastfeed the premature infant. Neonatal Netw 2006;25(2):77–86.

21. Yang CL, Kuo SC. [Assisting mother with preterm infant breastfeeding]. Hu Li Za Zhi 2007;54(4):61–6. Chinese.

22. Borrero-Pachón Mdel P, Olombrada-Valverde AE, Martínez de Alegría MI. Papel de la enfermería en el aternalo de la lactancia aternal en un recién nacido pretér-mino [Role of nursing in the development of breastfeeding in the premature newborn]. Enferm Clin 2010;20(2):119–25. Spanish.

23. Herber-Jonat S. Stillen beim Frühgeborenen [Breastfeeding in premature infants]. Z Geburtshilfe Neonatol 2007;211(1):8–12. German.

24. Dougherty D, Luther M. Birth to breast—a feeding care map for the NICU: helping the extremely low birth weight infant navigate the course. Neonatal Netw 2008; 27(6):371–7.

25. Briere CE, McGrath J, Cong X, et al. An integrative review of factors that influence breastfeeding duration for premature infants after NICU hospitalization. J Obstet Gynecol Neonatal Nurs 2014;43(3):272–81.

26. Giannì ML, Sannino P, Bezze E, et al. Does parental involvement affect the development of feeding skills in preterm infants? A prospective study. Early Hum Dev 2016;103:123–8.

27. Mörelius E, Kling K, Haraldsson E, et al. You can't flight, you need to fight-A qualitative study of mothers' experiences of feeding extremely preterm infants. J Clin Nurs 2020;29(13–14):2420–8.

Best Practices to Support Maternal Mental Health During the Transition from Neonatal Intensive Care Unit to Home: A Scoping Review

Jazmin D. Ramirez, BSN, RN[a],
Danielle Altares Sarik, PhD, APRN, CPNP-PC[b],*,
Yui Matsuda, PhD, PHNA-BC, MPH[a], Joy Ortiz, BSN, RN[c]

KEYWORDS

- Neonatal • NICU • Mental health • Transition of care • Hospital to home • Anxiety
- Depression • Postpartum

KEY POINTS

- Research has demonstrated that maternal mental health is a challenge for many mothers with infants who are hospitalized in the neonatal intensive care unit (NICU).
- Best practices to support maternal mental health during the period of transition from hospital to home include consistent, ongoing care, in-person support, and technology-based support.
- Addressing the mental well-being of the mother and ensuring proper support is a key aspect of the transition of care from the NICU to the home.

INTRODUCTION

In the United States, approximately 10% of births require admission into a neonatal intensive care unit (NICU) annually.[1] Most of the NICU admissions are due to prematurity, low birth weight, congenital anomalies, respiratory distress, or infections, and these conditions can be associated with a range of complex health concerns.[2] NICU admission and an infant's critical health condition are strongly linked to maternal psychological distress.[3–5] Parents of infants born prematurely are two times more

[a] University of Miami School of Nursing and Health Studies, 5030 Brunson Drive, Coral Gables, FL 33146, USA; [b] Nicklaus Children's Hospital, 3100 Southwest 62nd Avenue, Miami, FL 33155, USA; [c] Neonatal Intensive Care Unit, Nicklaus Children's Hospital, 3100 Southwest 62nd Avenue, Miami, FL 33155, USA
* Corresponding author. 3100 Southwest 62nd Avenue, Miami, FL 33155.
E-mail address: Danielle.sarik@nicklaushealth.org
Twitter: @DanielleSarik (D.A.S.)

Crit Care Nurs Clin N Am 36 (2024) 261–280
https://doi.org/10.1016/j.cnc.2023.11.006
0899-5885/24/© 2023 Elsevier Inc. All rights reserved.
ccnursing.theclinics.com

likely to experience depressive symptoms and other mental health challenges.[6] High levels of stress in mothers of premature infants have been correlated to elevated depressive, anxiety, and post-traumatic stress symptoms and negative maternal–infant attachment outcomes.[7–12] Subsequently, the impact of poor maternal mental health on maternal–infant attachment and parenting may have long-standing negative effects.[13]

In 2021, the US maternal mortality rate was 32.9 deaths per 100,000 live births, compared with 23.8 in 2020.[14] Owing to concerning increases in maternal mortality, Healthy People 2030 objectives include the reduction of maternal mortality as a leading health indicator.[15] An emerging leading cause of maternal mortality in the United States is self-harm,[16] which often occurs after mental health concerns. Mothers who give birth to infants admitted to an NICU are a markedly vulnerable population and disproportionately experience stress-related symptoms and mental health concerns, as compared with mothers who deliver healthy-term infants.[9,10,17,18] During the transition of discharge from the NICU to home, mothers may experience increased mental health concerns due to assuming responsibility for their infants' care after discharge and can have lower self-efficacy and higher stress at this time.[19]

Support for maternal mental health during the transition from the NICU to the home setting is key. Although some evidence-based interventions have demonstrated promise, no comprehensive review of the literature currently exists. Therefore, the purpose of this scoping review was to review best practices to support maternal mental health after discharge from the NICU setting in the acute period of transition from hospital to home.

METHODS

A scoping review was conducted to examine and synthesize the knowledge surrounding best practices to support maternal mental health after NICU discharge. According to Arksey and O'Malley[20] and later refined by Levac and colleagues[21] and Tricco and colleagues,[22] scoping reviews provide a systematic and rigorous approach to searching for and extracting data. Unlike systematic reviews, scoping reviews target identifying knowledge gaps, guiding decision-making, and setting research agendas and do not require formal evaluation of the quality of the studies. The consolidation of articles in this review allows for a critical appraisal of the practices and identification of gaps in care that can help guide future interventions to help support the mental health of mothers after NICU discharge.

A literature search was conducted to identify articles addressing best practices supporting maternal mental health post-NICU discharge. The electronic databases PubMed, CINHAL, and Psych Info were accessed for the search between January and March 2023. The assistance of a nursing science librarian was used to refine the search terms. Using Boolean operators and Subject Headings (eg, MeSH for PubMed) term finders, the following keywords were searched: "mental health," "anxiety," "depression," "stress," "mother," "NICU," "neonatal," "neonatal intensive care unit," "discharge," "post-NICU," "home," "intervention," and "resource."

Studies were included for final selection based on the following criteria: peer-reviewed articles published in the English language; publication within 10 years (2012–2023); available full text; focus on maternal mental health; address best practices or interventions after NICU discharge; and interventions available to patient and mother during the transition from hospital to home. The Preferred Reporting Items for Systematic Reviews and Meta-Analysis extension for Scoping Reviews recommendations were used as a guide for the methods of this review.[22]

Articles attained from the search were imported into Covidence,[23] a screening and data extraction tool, and were assessed for duplication. Titles and abstracts were evaluated by two independent reviewers (JR, DAS, YM) to identify those that appropriately addressed the review's objectives and met the inclusion criteria. Full texts of articles were then assessed for eligibility by two individual reviewers (JR, DAS, YM). Articles were excluded due to either wrong outcomes, intervention, or setting. All disagreements were resolved through team consultation (JR, DAS, YM) until a consensus was reached. Bibliographies from the attained articles were appraised and cross-referenced to ensure a comprehensive study search. A summary of the search process is illustrated in **Fig. 1**.

Pertinent data from each article that aligned with review objectives were extracted by one reviewer. The following data were extracted from each article: title, author, year of publication, country in which study was conducted, aim of study, study design, description of population, inclusion/exclusion criteria, total number of participants, instruments used, and key findings. A second reviewer examined the data extracted from each article to ascertain the accuracy, and a final data consensus was reached. A summary of the extracted data from each article is reported in **Table 1**.

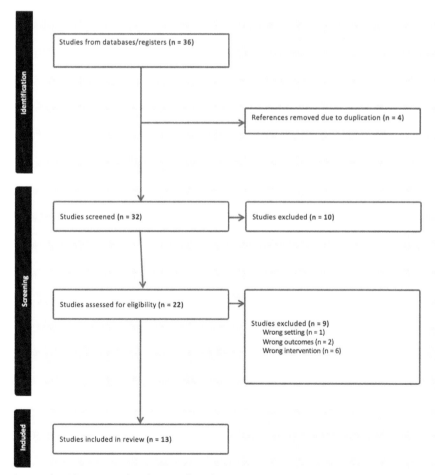

Fig. 1. Identification and inclusion of studies.

Table 1
Summary of extracted data from articles included in scoping review

Author, Year, Location	Aims/Purposes	Methods/Sample	Study Design	Instrument	Key Findings
Adama et al,[19] 2016 Australia	To synthesize qualitative studies regarding parents' experiences of caring for preterm infant at home after NICU discharge.	12 studies Parents who have cared for preterm infant at home after NICU discharge	Meta-synthesis	Qualitative studies	Nine categories were obtained from twelve qualitative studies and grouped into three syntheses: (1) support improves confidence in care; (2) dealing with challenges of caring for pre-term infant; and (3) overprotective parenting.
Adams et al,[24] 2022 United States	To identify if and why NICU families use online health communities (OHCs) and to assess how participation in these virtual spaces impacts relationships between parents and their child's medical team.	242 online survey participants; 176 Reddit posts NICU Parents	Quantitative and qualitative study (mixed method study)	Online survey and texts on an online platform, Reddit	58.3% ($n = 141$) of participants used specific social media sites or OHCs geared toward NICU parents and families to discuss their child in any way during their NICU stay. Stated reasons for using OHCs included: contacting other NICU families with similar problems (78%, $n = 110$), reducing anxiety regarding information given to me by my medical team (66.7%, $n = 94$), and sharing my successes with other NICU families with similar experiences at (63.1%, $n = 89$). Most of the participants noted an overall positive effect on communication, trust, and confidence with the medical team.

Baraldi et al,[26] 2020 Sweden	This study aimed to qualitatively explore the experience of parents of children born extremely preterm (EPT) in Sweden during the first year at home.	A total of 17 parents of 14 children born EPT were interviewed; eight parents were from the intervention group and nine parents from the control group in the Stockholm Preterm Interaction-Based Intervention, a post-discharge home visiting program.	Qualitative study	N/A	The main themes identified included: child-related concerns, parental inner states, and family dynamics. The main theme of child-related concerns had subthemes of continued medical concerns, child regulation difficulties, as well as incomplete recovery when coming home. The main theme of parental inner state had the subthemes of loneliness (both solitariness and alienation), ambivalent feelings (eg, the spectrum from relief to worry, from excitement to fear), and the process of keeping or letting go of a premature parental identity.
Breivold et al,[27] 2019 Norway	The aim of this study was to explore mothers' experiences after coming home from the hospital with a moderately to late preterm infant.	10 mothers with preterm infants	Qualitative study	N/A	Analysis yielded one main theme: "Seeing the light at the end of the tunnel" and four categories describing the mothers' experiences after coming home from hospital with a preterm

(continued on next page)

Table 1
(continued)

Author, Year, Location	Aims/Purposes	Methods/Sample	Study Design	Instrument	Key Findings
					infant. The categories included (1) finding a safe haven at home, (2) gaining support and learning to ensure optimal feeding, (3) seeing the child's possibilities, and (4) receiving professional attention and reassurance.
Fratantoni et al,[28] 2022 United States	To determine if peer support could improve parental mental health, including self-efficacy, stress, anxiety, and depression among NICU parents during the 12 mo after discharge.	300 English-speaking parents of infants who have stayed in NICU more than 2 wk	Randomized control trial	Perceived Stress Scale (PSS-10), Parental Stress Scale (PSS), Perceived Maternal Parenting Self-Efficacy Scale (PMPS-E), Center for Epidemiologic Studies Depression Scale (CES-D 10, CES-D 20)	Parental depression, anxiety, stress, and self-efficacy improved significantly for all participants, yet there were no differences between control (receive a care notebook) and intervention (care notebook plus peer support for 12 mo) groups. Infant ED visits, hospitalizations, immunization status, and developmental status at 12 mo did not differ between groups.

Garfield et al,[29] 2021 United States	To examine the trajectory of depression symptoms among mothers and fathers at several time points from NICU admission to 30 d after NICU discharge using the validated Edinburgh Postnatal Depression Scale (EPDS).	431 fathers and mothers of premature infants (<37 wk gestational age admitted to the NICU at Prentice Woman's Hospital, Chicago, Illinois)	Cohort study	Edinburgh Postnatal Depression Scale (EPDS), demographic survey	33% of mothers ($n = 57$) and 17% of fathers ($n = 21$) had a positive EPDS screening. Score change was 1.9 points different between mothers and fathers (confidence interval [CI]: 1.3–2.6; $P<.0001$), with mothers decreasing 2.9 points (CI: 2.1–3.7; $P<.0001$) and fathers decreasing 1.0 points (CI: 0.1–2.0; $P .04$) from the initial assessment to 30 d post-discharge. Over time, mothers' EPDS decreased 10.96 times (CI: 2.99–38.20; $P .0003$) and fathers' decreased at a nonsignificant rate. Admission or discharge screening improved 30-d depressive symptom prediction.
Gund et al,[30] 2013 Sweden	The aim of this randomized control study was to investigate whether the use of video conferencing or a Web application improves parents' satisfaction in taking care of a	34 families	Randomized control trial	Parent questionnaire and parent interviews	All parents in the web group found the Web application easy to use. Eighty-three percent of families stated it was good to have access to data through the application. All families

(continued on next page)

Table 1
(continued)

Author, Year, Location	Aims/Purposes	Methods/Sample	Study Design	Instrument	Key Findings
	premature infant at home and decreases the need for home visits.				in the video group found Skype easy to use and were satisfied with the video calls. Eighty-eight percent of the families reported that video calls were better than phone calls. Thirty-three percent of the families in the web group and 75% of those in the video group thought the need for home visits was decreased. Fifty percent of the families in the web group and 100% of those in the video reported that the intervention helped them to feel more confident in caring for their child.
Hawes et al,[31] 2016 United States	To examine maternal mental health, perceptions of readiness at NICU discharge, and social risk factors with depressive symptoms at 1 mo post-discharge in	734 mothers of 864 preterm infants	Cross-sectional study	Fragile Infant Parent Readiness Evaluation administered before discharge; the Edinburgh Postnatal Depression Scale	Mothers of early, moderate, and late preterm infants reported similar rates of possible depression (20%, 22%, and 18%, respectively) 1 mo after

	mothers of early (<32 wk), moderate (32–33 wk), and late (34–36 wk) preterm infants.			administered at 1 mo post-discharge	NICU discharge. History of mental health disorder, decreased perception of maternal well-being, decreased maternal comfort regarding infant, and decreased perception of family cohesion were associated with possible depression at 1 mo post-discharge.
Hedegaard Andersen et al,[25] 2021 Denmark	To determine whether the change from inpatient stays in NICU to offer neonatal homecare was associated with a reduced incidence rate of severe postpartum depression among mothers who gave birth prematurely.	46,456 mothers Nationwide Danish population registers (Pedersen, 2011), including the Medical Birth Register, Psychiatric Central Research Register (Mors et al, 2011), Danish National Prescription Registry (Kildemoes et al, 2011), National Patient Register (Lynge et al, 2011), and Statistics Denmark.	Cohort study	Measures of severe postpartum depression	Main findings demonstrate that implementation of neonatal homecare reduced the incidence rate of severe postpartum depression in mothers of preterm infants. Implementation yielded a 23% reduction, following the initial reduction incidence rates stabilized. Understanding the association between implementation of neonatal homecare and severe postpartum depression could contribute to the design of evidence-based interventions to prevent postpartum depression.

(continued on next page)

Table 1
(continued)

Author, Year, Location	Aims/Purposes	Methods/Sample	Study Design	Instrument	Key Findings
Horbar et al,[32] 2020 United States	To propose a more comprehensive approach that begins before birth and continues into childhood, involving health professionals, families, and communities as partners to meet the social as well as medical needs of infants and families.	N/A	Text and opinion	N/A	Mental health support listed as a potential better practice along with using home visits and ensuring links to community resources to improve transition to home experience.
Ji & Shim,[33] 2020 South Korea	To evaluate the efficacy of a community-based follow-up program on parenting stress, parenting efficacy, and coping among parents with premature infants.	56 mothers of premature infants who joined the infant service in Seoul, South Korea	Non-randomized experimental study	Parenting Stress Index (PSI), Parenting Sense of Competence (PSOC) scale for self-efficacy, and the Coping Health Inventory for Parents (CHIP)	Parents' coping behavior significantly differed in the experimental group (home visits by one experienced NICU nurse and one visiting nurse, 1–2 times a month for 6 mo and support group meetings) compared with the control group (two community visiting nurses, 1–2 times a month for 6 mo and support group meetings; $t = 3.14$, $P = .003$). In particular, coping subscale I, for maintaining the family

				situation ($t = 2.63$, $P = .011$), and subscale III, for understanding the infant's medical situation ($t = 4.30$, $P < .001$), showed significant differences in the experimental group. There were no significant between-group differences in parenting stress or parenting efficacy.
Khanjari et al,[34] 2021 Iran	Study aim was to investigate the effect of education through mobile health software on quality of life (QoL) and sense of coherence (SOC) of mothers with premature infants.	72 mothers with a premature infant	Non-randomized experimental study	Demographic questionnaire, SOC Scale, World Health Organization Quality of Life-BREF (WHOQoL-BREFW) Questionnaire	There were no statistically significant differences between groups in the QoL and SOC scores obtained in the pretest stage. For the intervention group, after the education, QoL and SOC scores significantly improved.

(continued on next page)

Table 1
(continued)

Author, Year, Location	Aims/Purposes	Methods/Sample	Study Design	Instrument	Key Findings
Kyno et al,[44] 2013	Study investigated differences in parents' experience of stress and concerns about caring for their premature child, based on participation in the Mother-Infant Transaction Program (MITP). Parental satisfaction with the intervention was also explored.	31 mothers of preterm infants	Qualitative research	Semistructured interview guide	Parents receiving the intervention reported that the knowledge, advice, guidance, and emotional support given during the intervention made them feel less stressed and more confident, competent, and secure caring for their premature child. Parents in the control group described feeling less involved and emotionally supported and reported more anxiety regarding development compared with parents in the intervention group. Parents in both groups reported high vigilance, monitoring of developmental milestones.

RESULTS

Study selection: Thirty-five articles were identified from a database and citation search. After review, 22 articles were excluded due to duplication, wrong interventions, design style, or outcomes. A total of 13 articles were included as part of the scoping review.[19,24–35]

Study characteristics: This scoping review yielded three qualitative studies, seven quantitative studies, one mixed method study, one meta-synthesis, and one text and opinion piece. Sample sizes ranged between 10 and 46,456 participants. Studies were conducted in Australia, Denmark, Iran, Norway, South Korea, Sweden, and the United States. Although the population of interest was mothers, studies that examined both mothers and fathers of NICU infants were also included. All studies included a discussion of interventions that occurred during the timeframe of post-NICU discharge. On reviewing the articles, three main categories of interventions regarding maternal mental health support were identified: (1) comprehensive evaluation of needs and continuity of care, (2) key role of in-person support, and (3) the potential to use technology-based support to increase mental health support. **Table 1** includes a summary of the extracted data from each article.

Comprehensive Evaluation of Needs and Continuity of Care

Initiatives aimed at converting interventions into practice and program planning require a thorough exploration of the needs of the target population.[36] Thus, 5 out of the 13 articles examined in this review advocated for the mental health support needs of mothers of NICU infants once discharged to home.[19,27,29,31,32] The need for consistent and ongoing care beginning from birth and extending through childhood that addressed the social, mental health, and medical needs of NICU infants and families was identified.[32] The risk of postpartum depression is similar for all NICU mothers regardless of infant gestational age at birth after NICU discharge.[31] Therefore, thorough parental mental health screening before NICU discharge along with training of NICU bedside staff to help identify and communicate with parents encountering mental health challenges was highlighted as a pivotal component of the continuum of care.[29] Factors such as the history of mental illness, perceived lack of social support system/family cohesion, and lack of confidence in the ability to provide care (perception of readiness at NICU discharge) were identified as potential indicators of the need for enhanced mental health support post-NICU discharge.[31]

A potential better practice addressed by Horbar and colleagues included mental health support for caregivers via the utilization of home visits and ensuring links to community resources to improve the transition from NICU to home.[32] Two articles used a qualitative approach to report on parents' experience caring for preterm infants at home after NICU discharge.[19,27] The day of discharge from the NICU was reported to be received with mixed emotions, a time of joy and uncertainty/fear. Parents expressed distress regarding the responsibility of caring for their infants alone at home due to a perceived lack of knowledge of infant care tasks and infants' medical history. They reported feelings of fear, delayed joy in motherhood, need for support, guilt, and weakened confidence. With well-managed parental support rooted in thorough needs assessment starting in the NICU and continuing after discharge, it is anticipated that mothers' confidence in their ability to provide care and cope with parental stressors may be improved.[19] Apart from having a strong social support system, Breivold and colleagues also stressed the importance NICU mothers gave to having a good relationship with their own health care provider in order to share concerns surrounding their mental health.[27] Continuity of care between NICU health care providers and community resources is an essential component to improving maternal mental health outcomes and its cascading effect on the family and infant well-being post-NICU discharge.

In-person Support

An essential mode of mental health support addressed in this review involved in-person support and communication. Although in-person support can occur in many forms, some of the methods discussed included NICU peer support groups, neonatal home-care, community-based follow-up programs, and pre- and post-hospitalization interventions seeking to bridge the transition to home (eg, Mother-Infant Transaction Program [MITP]). Five out of the thirteen articles used person-to-person interventions for maternal mental health support.[25,26,28,33,35] The findings of a study investigating the effects of having an NICU peer navigator as a resource to parents during NICU stay and up to 12 months post-discharge showed no difference between control and intervention groups regarding parental depression, anxiety, stress, self-efficacy, and infant care utilization as both groups improved significantly.[28] One potential limitation was that peer support was presented at discharge, a busy time for NICU parents as they are preparing for their transition. Therefore, introductions to peer support earlier on during NICU stay may have been better received by parents to build relationships and trust, potentially having a more positive effect on maternal mental health outcomes.[28]

Another study analyzed the association between neonatal home care and post-partum depression.[25] Heegaard Anderson and colleagues conducted a register-based, population-wide study of all mothers who gave birth prematurely from 1994 to 2017 and whose infants spent at least one night in the NICU.[25] The implementation of neonatal homecare was associated with a 23% reduction in postpartum depression. In-person neonatal homecare post-NICU discharge was therefore identified as a highly effective intervention for reducing postpartum depression in mothers.[25] Further, a study evaluating the efficacy of a community-based follow-up program on parenting stress, parenting efficacy, and coping among parents with premature infants was included in this review.[33] The intervention consisted of structured home visits and self-help group meetings for 6 months. Participants in the intervention group received visits by an experienced NICU nurse and the control group received a visit from a nonspecialized nurse. Parenting coping behavior was significantly better in the intervention group when compared with the control. However, parenting stress and self-efficacy did not differ between groups. Parenting stress was reduced in both groups after home visits, providing some evidence for the role of in-person support.[33]

Baraldi and colleagues explored and compared parent's experiences during the first year after NICU discharge, exploring differences between those who did and did not receive post-discharge intervention.[26] In addition, the perception of participating in a home visiting program was evaluated. Parents addressed feelings of loneliness, worry, fear, and stress as well as the lack of adequate support for babies' special conditions. These results highlight the need for mental health assessments once home from NICU. In Sweden where this study was conducted, preterm infants being discharged with feeding tubes or supplementary oxygen received 3 months of at-home nurse visits to support and monitor additional medical needs post-discharge. Furthermore, the parents of infants who did not require feeding or oxygen support felt a sense of security and a decrease in worry due to participation in the study's intervention group and receiving 10 neonatal nurse-led homecare visits throughout the first year after discharge. This finding supports the positive impact of in-person psychosocial support for parents of NICU infants after discharge.[26]

A separate study investigated an early intervention program, the MITP. The main aim of the MITP was to teach parents how to be sensitive and responsive to their infant's cues, to reduce both the infants' and parents' stress and to enhance child development and parental adjustment.[35] The program was composed of eleven 1-hour sessions with each parent and child. Parents who participated in the intervention reported that the knowledge, advice, and emotional support given during the intervention made them feel less stressed and more confident. Control group participants reported feeling less involved, less emotionally supported, and more anxious. The investigators concluded that in-person education and training is an effective form of mental health support for parents of NICU infants transitioning to home.

Technology-Based Support

Technology-based programs and applications have grown in popularity and use in recent years. Three articles addressed technology-based mental health support interventions for mothers of NICU infants post-discharge. Interventions included the use of online health communities (OHCs), video conferencing or Web applications, and mobile health software.[24,30,34] Adams and colleagues aimed to identify if and why NICU families (242 participants) used OHCs and assessed whether the use of such online resources impacted the relationship between parents and their child's medical team. A large percentage of parents (66.7%) used OHCs to reduce anxiety regarding medical information given to them by providers, and the majority (78%) wanted to connect with other parents to decrease feelings of loneliness. The use of OHCs did not negatively impact parents' relationship with their child's medical team.[24] Therefore, there is evidence that the use of such OHCs may provide mental health support without negatively impacting the medical team and parents' relationships.

Video conferencing, or telehealth, is a popular alternative to home visits or doctors' visits for mothers of NICU graduates.[30] A randomized control study investigated the usefulness and receptiveness of parents using video conferencing or Web applications in place of in-person home visits and found that parents reported high satisfaction with video conferencing. Eighty-eight percent of parents reported that video calls were a better alternative than traditional phone calls, and 50% of families expressed that video calls were less stressful than home visits.[30] Therefore, telehealth may provide a means of supporting mothers during the transition from hospital to home which is both satisfactory and may also be less stressful.

Kahnjari and colleagues examined mothers' quality of life (QoL) and sense of coherence (SOC), of which maternal confidence is a subscale, after participating in a 3-month education program through mobile health software.[34] Both the control and intervention groups had the software installed on their smartphones; however, only the intervention group had access to all educational content. On analysis, participants in the intervention group had significantly improved post-test QoL and SOC scores when compared with the control group.[34] This study highlighted the benefits that mobile health programs may provide mothers of NICU infants once home, supporting overall mental health.

DISCUSSION

After reviewing identified articles and outcomes, three major areas of evidence-based support for maternal mental health during the transition from the NICU to home were identified. The major themes that emerged were (1) comprehensive evaluation of needs and continuity of care, (2) the key role of in-person support, and (3) the potential to use technology-based support to increase mental health support.

Our scoping review results illustrated that successful mental health support for the maternal population during the critical time transitioning from the NICU to home requires careful consideration beginning during the NICU stay.[31] Thorough and routine mental health screenings for these mothers before discharge by trained staff can support mothers of NICU infants to make a successful transition to home, enhancing the chances for their optimal post-discharge mental health.[37] NICU nurses are at infants' bedside to provide care, and with appropriate training, NICU nurses could be instrumental in supporting mothers' mental health, screening for mental health symptoms, and making referrals as indicated.[38] Optimizing maternal mental health facilitates mothers to not only provide their infants' basic needs but also continue bonding with the infants, ultimately promoting their optimal health outcomes and infant mental health.[39,40]

The availability of both in-person and technology-based support also emerged as a key theme in supporting the mental health of mothers during the hospital-to-home transition. Several of the articles reviewed identified having a form of post-discharge support, whether home visits,[25,33] video conferencing with health care providers,[30] or access to peer support groups[28] as beneficial. Peer support for mothers beginning in the NICU and ideally continuing during the transition to home and community may ease the transition and support post-discharge maternal mental health.

Once discharged to home, mental health support should continue with close follow-up of NICU mothers and their infants. The literature demonstrates that coordinated home visits by experienced NICU nurses provide valuable support and increase mothers' confidence in caring for their infant, decrease anxiety, and strengthen coping behaviors.[33] These visits optimally should include surveying parents' perceptions of their child and addressing concerns that may arise from miscommunication, lack of communication, and availability of providers as well as the general comfort of mothers in communicating with the medical team which often includes multiple providers. Post-discharge support may also be enhanced by several services that appeal to a range of mothers' educational, coping, and mental health needs. The use of social media and technology helps with this goal. Video conferencing with health care providers was better received by mothers than conventional phone calls. Peer support groups continuing online after discharge were also found to enhance optimal maternal mental health. Post-discharge support using technology-based education is also not to be overlooked. Parents introduced to OHCs have decreased anxiety regarding caring for their child after discharge. Of note, participation in these communities was not shown to negatively impact the mother's relationship with their child's medical team. Mobile health software available for use anytime on smartphones was also a technology that enhanced mothers' coping and eased concerns.

The use of technology to provide connection and support to mothers as they transition from the NICU to home also emerged as an important consideration. Although in-person services may not be readily available to mothers in remote settings, geographic challenges can be addressed through technology, such as the use of applications, telehealth platforms, or online peer support groups. These methods can allow mothers to access support systems in a nontraditional way during the post-NICU transition period. In addition, programs that use telehealth or video applications to provide transition-of-care support for caregivers of infants discharged from the NICU may offer a template for meaningful support and mental health surveillance.[41,42]

Practice Implications

Although some investigation of interventions during hospitalization that may impact mental health exists, evidence has only demonstrated a modest impact on maternal distress.[43] Successful support for this vulnerable mother–child population likely requires careful consideration of the mothers' mental health beginning during the NICU stay and continuing into the home and community setting. Research suggests that maternal mental health is highly vulnerable during the transition to home from the NICU [19,27,29,32] which is a period in which clinicians must actively intervene to provide support, decrease mortality, morbidity, and self-harm, and facilitate optimal infant health and developmental outcomes.

Future Directions

Despite the clear understanding that many mothers are facing a mental health crisis, there is little agreement about how best to address this issue. For those mothers with an infant hospitalized in the NICU, mental health concerns are compounded. Although these trends have been well documented, little has been published on the unique mental health trajectory and needs of mothers after their infant is discharged from the NICU. As clinicians, it is important that we recognize the transition of care from hospital to home as a particularly vulnerable time for mothers and act appropriately. Studies that investigate supportive approaches should be conducted in a scientifically rigorous way, including randomized controlled trials where appropriate, to assess the impact of evidence-based interventions.

Limitations

One of the inherent limitations in this scoping review is the inclusion of studies only written and available in the English language. This may have limited the cultural diversity of the interventions reviewed. In addition, as we focused on maternal mental health, we may have excluded articles focused on fathers or other family members that would be of value to review.

SUMMARY

Mothers with an infant hospitalized in the NICU are at an increased risk of mental health concerns, including depression and anxiety. Successful mental health support during the critical time of transition from hospital to home requires careful consideration of the mothers' mental health beginning during the NICU stay with continuity of care as they transition to the home and community setting. Major themes from a scoping review to identify best practices to support maternal mental health include (1) comprehensive evaluation of needs and continuity of care, (2) key role of in-person support, and (3) the potential to use technology-based support to increase mental health support.

CLINICS CARE POINTS

- Mothers with an infant hospitalized in the neonatal intensive care unit (NICU) are at an increased risk of mental health concerns, including depression and anxiety.
  - Factors that may contribute to increased mental health concerns include postpartum depression and anxiety surrounding their infant's health and follow-up care needs, decreased opportunities for maternal-infant attachment, and adjustment to a reality that differs from what was planned.
- Successful mental health support during the critical time of transition from hospital to home requires careful consideration of the mother's mental health and needs beginning during the NICU stay.
- A scoping review based on 13 articles was conducted to identify best practices for maternal mental health during the transition from the NICU to home and found the following:[19,24–35]

- There is a need for consistent and ongoing care beginning from birth and extending to childhood that addresses the social, mental health, and medical needs of NICU infants and families.[32]
- In-person support and communication, including NICU peer support groups, neonatal homecare, community-based follow-up programs, and pre-post hospitalization interventions seeking to bridge the transition to home, should be offered or implemented.
- Technology-based support, such as telehealth or online support groups, can provide an alternative to mothers with geographic limitations in access to care.

DISCLOSURE

The authors have no conflicts of interest to disclose.

REFERENCES

1. Braun D, Braun E, Chiu V, et al. Trends in neonatal intensive care unit utilization in a large integrated health care system. JAMA Netw Open 2020;3(6):e205239.
2. Center for Disease Control and Prevention (CDC). Reproductive Health: Preterm Birth. Published online 2022. Available at: https://www.cdc.gov/reproductive-health/maternalinfanthealth/pretermbirth.htm#print. Accessed July 28, 2023.
3. Roque ATF, Lasiuk GC, Radünz V, et al. Scoping review of the mental health of parents of infants in the NICU. J Obstet Gynecol Neonatal Nurs 2017;46(4): 576–87.
4. Kestler-Peleg M, Stenger V, Lavenda O, et al. "I'll Be There": informal and formal support systems and mothers' psychological distress during NICU hospitalization. Children 2022;9(12). https://doi.org/10.3390/children9121958.
5. Dubner SE, Morales MC, Marchman VA, et al. Maternal mental health and engagement in developmental care activities with preterm infants in the NICU. J Perinatol 2023;43(7):871–6.
6. Deshwali A, Dadhwal V, Vanamail P, et al. Prevalence of mental health problems in mothers of preterm infants admitted to NICU: a cross-sectional study. Int J Gynecol Obstet 2023;160(3):1012–9.
7. Bonacquisti A, Geller PA, Patterson CA. Maternal depression, anxiety, stress, and maternal-infant attachment in the neonatal intensive care unit. J Reprod Infant Psychol 2020;38(3):297–310.
8. Gerstein ED, Njoroge WFM, Paul RA, et al. Maternal depression and stress in the neonatal intensive care unit: associations with mother–child interactions at age 5 years. J Am Acad Child Adolesc Psychiatry 2019;58(3):350–8.e2.
9. Holditch-Davis D, Miles MS, Weaver MA, et al. Patterns of distress in African-American mothers of preterm infants. J Dev Behav Pediatr 2009;30(3):193–205.
10. Misund AR, Nerdrum P, Diseth TH. Mental health in women experiencing preterm birth. BMC Pregnancy Childbirth 2014;14(1):263.
11. Salomè S, Mansi G, Lambiase CV, et al. Impact of psychological distress and psychophysical wellbeing on posttraumatic symptoms in parents of preterm infants after NICU discharge. Ital J Pediatr 2022;48(1):13.
12. Shelton S, Meaney-Delman D, Hunter M, et al. Depressive symptoms and the relationship of stress, sleep, and well-being among NICU mothers. J Nurs Educ Pract 2014;4:70–9.
13. Goodman SH, Rouse MH, Connell AM, et al. Maternal depression and child psychopathology: a meta-analytic review. Clin Child Fam Psychol Rev 2011; 14(1):1–27.

14. Hoyert D.L. Maternal mortality rate in the United States, 2021, 2023, NCHS Health E-Stats. https://www.cdc.gov/nchs/data/hestat/maternal-mortality/2021/maternal-mortality-rates-2021.htm.

15. Healthy People 2030, National vital statistics system (NVSS-M). Center for Disease Control and Prevention; 2018. https://health.gov/healthypeople/objectives-and-data/browse-objectives/pregnancy-and-childbirth/reduce-maternal-deaths-mich-04.

16. Collier A, ris Y, Molina RL. Maternal mortality in the United States: updates on trends, causes, and solutions. NeoReviews 2019;20(10):e561–74.

17. Jubinville J, Newburn-Cook C, Hegadoren K, Lacaze-Masmonteil T. Symptoms of acute stress disorder in mothers of premature infants. Adv Neonatal Care 2012; 12(4):246–53.

18. Miles MS, Funk SG, Kasper MA. The neonatal intensive care unit environment: sources of stress for parents. AACN Adv Crit Care 1991;2(2):346–54.

19. Adama EA, Bayes S, Sundin D. Parents' experiences of caring for preterm infants after discharge from Neonatal Intensive Care Unit: a meta-synthesis of the literature. J Neonatal Nurs 2016;22(1):27–51.

20. Arksey H, O'Malley L. Scoping studies: towards a methodological framework. Int J Soc Res Methodol 2005;8(1):19–32.

21. Levac D, Colquhoun H, O'Brien KK. Scoping studies: advancing the methodology. Implement Sci 2010;5(1):69.

22. Tricco AC, Lillie E, Zarin W, et al. PRISMA extension for scoping reviews (PRISMA-ScR): checklist and explanation. Ann Intern Med 2018;169(7):467–73.

23. Covidence systematic review software. Published online Updated 2022.

24. Adams SY, Tucker R, Lechner BE. The new normal: parental use of online health communities in the NICU. Pediatr Res 2022;91(7):1827–33.

25. Andersen KSH, Holm KG, Nordentoft M, et al. Association between neonatal homecare for preterm infants and incidence of severe postpartum depression in mothers. J Affect Disord 2021;278:453–9.

26. Baraldi E, Allodi MW, Smedler AC, et al. Parents' experiences of the first year at home with an infant born extremely preterm with and without post-discharge intervention: ambivalence, loneliness, and relationship impact. Int J Environ Res Public Health 2020;17(24). https://doi.org/10.3390/ijerph17249326.

27. Breivold K, Hjaelmhult E, Sjöström-Strand A, et al. Mothers' experiences after coming home from the hospital with a moderately to late preterm infant – a qualitative study. Scand J Caring Sci 2019;33(3):632–40.

28. Fratantoni K, Soghier L, Kritikos K, et al. Giving parents support: a randomized trial of peer support for parents after NICU discharge. J Perinatol 2022;42(6): 730–7.

29. Garfield CF, Lee YS, Warner-Shifflett L, et al. Maternal and paternal depression symptoms during NICU stay and transition home. Pediatrics 2021;148(2). e2020042747.

30. Gund A, Sjöqvist BA, Wigert H, et al. A randomized controlled study about the use of eHealth in the home health care of premature infants. BMC Med Inform Decis Mak 2013;13(1):22.

31. Hawes K, McGowan E, O'Donnell M, et al. Social emotional factors increase risk of postpartum depression in mothers of preterm infants. J Pediatr 2016;179:61–7.

32. Horbar JD, Edwards EM, Ogbolu Y. Our responsibility to follow through for NICU infants and their families. Pediatrics 2020;146(6):e20200360.

33. Ji Eun Sun Shim Ka Ka, Shim KK. Effects of a community-based follow-up program for parents with premature infants on parenting stress, parenting efficacy, and coping. Child Health Nurs Res 2020;26(3):366–75.

34. Khanjari S, Bell EF, Sadeghi LA, et al. The impact of a mobile health intervention on the sense of coherence and quality of life of mothers with premature infants. J Neonatal Nurs 2021;27(6):444–50.

35. Kynø NM, Ravn IH, Lindemann R, et al. Parents of preterm-born children; sources of stress and worry and experiences with an early intervention programme – a qualitative study. BMC Nurs 2013;12(1):28.

36. Bartholomew LK, Parcel GS, Kok G. Intervention mapping: a process for developing theory and evidence-based health education programs. Health Educ Behav 1998;25(5):545–63.

37. Bernardo J, Rent S, Arias-Shah A, et al. Parental stress and mental health symptoms in the NICU: recognition and interventions. NeoReviews 2021;22(8): e496–505.

38. Grunberg VA, Geller PA, Hoffman C, et al. Parental mental health screening in the NICU: a psychosocial team initiative. J Perinatol 2022;42(3):401–9.

39. Goodman JH. Perinatal depression and infant mental health. Arch Psychiatr Nurs 2019;33(3):217–24.

40. Runkle JD, Risley K, Roy M, et al. Association between perinatal mental health and pregnancy and neonatal complications: a retrospective birth cohort study. Wom Health Issues 2023;33(3):289–99.

41. Sarik DA, Matsuda Y, Terrell EA, et al. A telehealth nursing intervention to improve the transition from the neonatal intensive care unit to home for infants & caregivers: preliminary evaluation. J Pediatr Nurs 2022;67:139–47.

42. Sarik DA, Matsuda Y, Betz CL. Baby steps: improving the transition from hospital to home for neonatal patients and caregivers through a nurse-led telehealth program. In: *Worldwide successful pediatric nurse-led models of care*. 1st edition. Springer; 2023. https://link.springer.com/book/10.1007/978-3-031-22152-1.

43. Sabnis A, Fojo S, Nayak SS, et al. Reducing parental trauma and stress in neonatal intensive care: systematic review and meta-analysis of hospital interventions. J Perinatol 2019;39(3):375–86.

44. Kynø NM, Ravn IH, Lindemann R, et al. Parents of preterm-born children; sources of stress and worry and experiences with an early intervention programme - a qualitative study. BMC Nurs 2013;12(1):28.

Legacy Building

The Experience of Heartbeat Recordings for Bereaved Caregivers in Pediatrics

Nicole Polara, MMT, MT-BC

KEYWORDS

- Legacy building • Memory making • Music therapy • Bereavement
- Continuing bonds • Caregivers • Parents • Heartbeat recording

KEY POINTS

- The reader will learn of the potential impact losing a child has on a parent or caregiver.
- The reader will gain an understanding of how music therapy can support patients and families at the end of life through heartbeat recordings.
- The reader will gain insight into the use of heartbeat recordings in anticipatory grief in parents of children nearing the end of life.

INTRODUCTION

Bereavement is understood as both an event of loss as well as adjusting to said loss. According to the Center for Fatality Review and Prevention, almost 40,000 children in the United States lose their lives each year, with sudden and unidentified infant deaths and medical-related deaths being two of the highest causes (2020).[1] The death of a child is a special sorrow. No matter the circumstances, a child's death is a life-altering experience and is one of the greatest stressors a person can endure, according to the Institute of Health (2003).[2] In addition to the stress, parents may also suffer from social and economic challenges, depressive symptoms, poor well-being, health complications, marital issues, mental health challenges, and even premature death for both mothers and fathers.[3] Parents and caretakers of infants have experienced chronic sorrow, a prolonged, recurrent, and pervasive sadness related to grief and loss.

In a selection by Siegal,[4] a group of bereaved parents define grief as unquantifiable, no matter what age the child is when they die. Parents in this group described that gathering records of their child's life served an important role in creating and sustaining a continuing bond. Parents also felt comfort in doing "normal" tasks with their child, even after death. This included bathing them, dressing them, holding them,

Department of Child Life and Integrative Care, Cincinnati Children's Hospital Medical Center, 3333 Burnet Avenue, MLC 5003, Cincinnati, OH 45229, USA
E-mail address: nicole.polara@cchmc.org

Crit Care Nurs Clin N Am 36 (2024) 281–287
https://doi.org/10.1016/j.cnc.2023.11.007
0899-5885/24/Published by Elsevier Inc.

and some even took their child home after the death. These experiences allowed the parents to feel like "normal" parents and have peaceful moments with their child, outside of the commotion and hustle of a neonatal intensive care unit (NICU).

Although the opportunity for memory making and creating a foundation for continuing bonds exists in so many ways, there are still immense struggles with the physicality of loss for these parents. Parents and caregivers look for tangible items that contain their infant's scent and touch such as clothes and blankets. However, over time, these sensory comforts begin to fade, and because their time spent together is so short, the parents are left with little material items or treasures from their child. Legacy-building opportunities provided by hospitals include hand and footprint molds as a memento, or cards that were written by family members and staff, that may help parents and caregivers cope with their loss. Heartbeat recordings are another way to offer parents a material item or treasure.. They can hold these recordings or other mementos close or share them with family and friends to sustain the continuing bond that has hopefully been created.

Experts on bereavement and grief rely on the continuing bonds theory to help individuals cope and live with the chronic sorrow and tragedy that accompanies loss. Continuing bonds theory is widely used to help understand the grieving process. This theory shares the idea of creating and maintaining a connection with a deceased loved one. Klass and Steffen[5] write, "Making meaning is making sense of the events leading to the death and around the death, making sense of our relationship to the deceased, and making sense of our ongoing lives after death."[(p8)] A continuing bond is an idea or a feeling that may manifest in bereaved individuals in different ways. Continuing bonds in practice may focus on the relationship with the deceased while the bereaved are expected to coexist and cope with the demands of their own life. Individuals may have the opportunity to create a legacy, or a parent, caregiver, or family member may do this for them. A legacy allows one's life story to live on through items such as a lock of hair, hand molds, handprints, photographs, artwork, and heartbeat recordings. In many pediatric hospitals in the United States, these legacy items are offered to help families who are experiencing anticipatory grief, loss, and bereavement.

Boles and Jones conducted a systematic review of 67 quantitative and qualitative studies that describe legacy perceptions and interventions in pediatric and adult palliative care recipients. As the first systematic review, this paper synthesized implications for practice, theory, and policy on legacy-building experiences. There was consistency found across studies defining notions of legacy as sharing of oneself, stories, or belongings from one to another, a meaning-making process, and a vehicle for being remembered.[6(p545)] The authors conclude that the concept of legacy as an intervention or therapeutic goal is feasible for adult and pediatric patients and may make modest improvements in symptom-related stress and well-being. The concept of legacy also applies to neonatal patients and infants.

Legacy-building experiences or memory items have become increasingly common in supporting anticipatory grief in loss and bereavement throughout hospital settings. Schaefer and colleagues[7] qualitatively explored legacy artwork, including paintings, graffiti collages, plaster sculptures, and wall murals with bereaved parents who participated in these experiences with their child before their death from cancer. Five themes emerged from the interview concluding that creating legacy artwork facilitates family bonding and memory making and opens communication between family members, provides opportunities for parents to engage in life review and the meaning of their child's death, ameliorates parents' grief after their child's death, and may also reduce compassion fatigue in health-care providers. The connection between legacy-making and continuing bonds is made here as parents reported feelings of comfort and connection with their child through this artwork because it included their handprints, preferences, and signatures, all of which are unique to their child. Parents and health-care providers also report that legacy artwork should be offered as early as possible with the intent to capture the child's illness journey rather than solely capturing end of life. The results and emergent themes suggest that legacy artwork provides great benefits for bereaved parents, as well as creating global meaning by retelling the stories about the lives of their children.

Because legacy-building experiences, such as artwork, hand molds, locks of hair, and so forth, have been researched and suggested as beneficial in bereavement, there has been an increased interest in heartbeat recordings for anticipatory grief and bereavement for caregivers in pediatric and neonatal medical settings. This intervention, created by board-certified music therapist Brian Schreck at Cincinnati Children's Hospital Medical Center,[8] involves audio recording the patient's heartbeat or other respiratory sounds with a digital stethoscope to construct and preserve the patient's legacy, as well as acts as a therapeutic tool. In collaboration with the patient and/or family, recorded or live music can be combined with the heartbeat while preserving the integrity of the patient's heartbeat recording to create an opportunity for memory-making or legacy-building.

According to the American Music Therapy Association,[9,10] "music therapy is the clinical and evidence-based use of music interventions to accomplish individualized goals within a therapeutic relationship by a credentialed professional who has completed an approved music therapy program." In the pediatric medical setting, music therapy is used to promote healthy coping skills, pain management, autonomy, and psychosocial well-being during hospitalization and medical treatment.[11] At the end of life, music therapists can help support anticipatory grief and bereavement through heartbeat recording interventions.

Current research on heartbeat recordings focuses on the experiences of patients and caregivers during the recording process within the palliative care setting. Schreck and Economos[12] use case examples to explore heartbeat recording and composing in perinatal palliative care and hospice care. Schreck and Economos[12] state, "This process aims to capture moments in time, which may be preserved for future connection with the patient and family."[(p22)] The authors of this study conclude that the strength of heartbeat recordings in perinatal palliative care relies heavily on the therapeutic relationship between the music therapist and the patient and/or family.

Similarly, Walden and colleagues[13] interviewed parents of children with progressive neurogenerative illnesses to explore the lived experiences of heartbeat recordings for these parents and found that heartbeat recordings lead to meaning-making experiences that validate the child's existence. The authors also found that heartbeat recordings supported parents' expression of grief and their ability to cope. Walden and colleagues[13] also suggest further research with diverse populations to validate this research.

Additionally, a study by Corrigan and colleagues[14] analyzed the use of heartbeat recordings in a different setting to promote mother–infant bonding in the NICU. Family-centered care has been adopted in many NICUs to encourage family members to play a more active role in their infant's care. In this study, the authors used heartbeat recordings to help parents bond with their infant, as well as an intervention for support to infants undergoing uncomfortable procedures. In this study, heartbeat recordings were not necessarily used palliatively; however, it seems the emphasis of the heartbeat recordings was still reliant on the therapeutic relationship.

Findings from a preliminary study about the experience of heartbeat recordings for bereaved parents of hospitalized pediatric patients suggest that although the heartbeat recording may be difficult to listen to, especially at the beginning, parents are still grateful for the recording and comforted by it.[15] Parents also shared that listening to the heartbeat recording brought them positive feelings such as joy, and although it was very emotional, it was also treasured. Parents in this study also described that the heartbeat recording was meaningful to them because it elicited positive memories and a sense of still being with their child. Parents and caregivers in this study shared that they have used their heartbeat recordings at memorial services, in video tributes, and slide shows, and have been put inside stuffed animals. A Likert scale from this preliminary study displayed parents' overall experience with heartbeat recordings.

Although some patients and caregivers create heartbeat recordings in collaboration with the music therapist throughout their treatment, others have not had this relationship but are, nevertheless, provided with heartbeat recordings during a one-time interaction with a music therapist. Preliminary research suggests that receiving this recording in the absence of a collaborative relationship with the music therapist may not provide optimum conditions to derive positive effects from the legacy. "Although families appreciate having a physical product to cherish, the strength in this intervention lies in its flexibility to be offered as a process within the context of a music therapy relationship."[12(p24)] In practice, heartbeat recordings are offered to patients and families, whether or not they have received music therapy services throughout the course of their child's treatment. However, research on the experience of heartbeat recordings for bereaved caregivers does not exist outside of the context of the therapeutic relationship. To maintain the integrity and therapeutic value of heartbeat recordings, it is essential for music therapists and health-care providers to understand the impact that heartbeat recordings have on bereaved caregivers with diverse experiences.

DISCUSSION

The sound of a child's heartbeat is, if not the first, one of the first sounds a mother or caregiver hears when the child is in utero. This sound is unique to their child and is one of the first aspects of identity that is manifested by an individual. The sound of someone's heartbeat is an intimate sign of life. Often the heartbeat is the first and last sound a parent or caregiver hears of their loved one. Having, listening to, and using a heartbeat recording, whether it be with or without music, may be a bittersweet experience for bereaved caregivers. The sound of the heartbeat holds varying emotions, memories, and sensations throughout the bereavement process, which is why a heartbeat recording may be such a strong continuing bond for bereaved parents and caregivers.

Heartbeat recordings create a sense of connectedness in being with the deceased and may assist parents or caregivers in developing a healthy continuing bond. A continuing bond is an aid in the grieving process that allows bereaved individuals to have a relationship with their deceased loved one. A heartbeat recording may be considered a continuing bond with its ability to provide a unique and special sound or song for the bereaved. Continuing bonds may also assist in helping individuals cope with chronic sorrow. Because the sound of the heartbeat is a sign of life, it may allow bereaved parents or caregivers to feel as though their loved one is still there with them. Therefore, heartbeat recordings may bring a sense of comfort and joy because they help bereaved caregivers to feel as though they are not gone because they can still hear the beating of their loved one's heart. The heartbeat recording, as a continuing bond, helps bereaved caregivers remember the legacy of their loved one and helps them remember how special and unique they were. It helps them to not forget the impact they have left on their own lives and the lives of others, even if they were only physical with them for a short period.

When music therapists begin the process of creating a heartbeat recording, they begin by inviting patients, if old enough, and/or caregivers/parents to share wishes about the legacy that is to be created. Creating this continuing bond with their loved one starts with a conversation about their memories and a discussion about how they can preserve their child's legacy. When patients and families are offered a heartbeat recording, they can choose whether they would prefer music added to it or not. The music can be prerecorded, or it can be music that has been recreated by the music therapist or even by a patient or family member. According to Love and colleagues,[16] all patients and families should be offered the same legacy-building and memory-making opportunities at the end of life. Therefore, music therapists should offer the addition of music whether or not they have had multiple sessions or only one session with a patient and/or family.

Schreck and Economos[12] found that the therapeutic relationship with a music therapist is highly valued and is what strengthens the heartbeat recording intervention. Although the impact of having a relationship with a music therapist before receiving a heartbeat recording is still understudied, it has been suggested that parents and caregivers who have a larger role in creating the recording, or who had more interactions with a music therapist, may have an enhanced experience with their heartbeat recording, increasing the therapeutic value during anticipatory grief and bereavement. Having a previous relationship with the music therapist, as well as the experience of having creative input into the recording process, may also have a direct impact on parents' and caregivers' use of their loved one's heartbeat recording, increasing its usefulness in creating a sustainable continuing bond in their bereavement process.

Research on heartbeat recordings is limited; however, it is used regularly in pediatric hospitals. Consideration needs to be placed on the timing of introducing heartbeat recordings to families, who will introduce the heartbeat recording to a family, and when a heartbeat recording is completed. Presumably, it is more beneficial to introduce and begin the heartbeat recording process with a family sooner rather than later, in order to ensure a therapeutic relationship between the music therapist and family. However, in practice, it is common that a patient may decompensate quickly causing the music therapist to urgently perform a heartbeat recording. It is essential for health-care providers to understand the intimacy and impact that heartbeat recordings have because, possibly, this could be the last sound of life that the family has of their loved one.

The introduction and initiation of the heartbeat recording project must be done with care and compassion. Because of the use of technology involved in these recordings, it is recommended that a trained music therapist facilitate the intervention to maintain the therapeutic value and integrity of the heartbeat recording. Another consideration that should be taken is that not every patient is an appropriate candidate for a heartbeat recording. For example, if a patient is on an oscillator ventilator, the digital stethoscope may not pick up the patient's actual heartbeat. Religious or spiritual implications should also be considered. A specially trained music therapist should always be consulted before offering this intervention to a family.

Although heartbeat recordings have historically been a palliative care intervention, heartbeat recordings may be introduced and used as a commemorative item for a patient and a family's hospitalization journey. A heartbeat recording may be done at any time to help create a patient's legacy, even if they are not nearing end of life or have a better prognosis. Creating a heartbeat recording with a music therapist may provide a patient and family with a positive memento to take away from their otherwise potentially stressful hospital experience. This intervention is frequently used in the NICU as a way to promote healthy bonding between the parents or caregiver and their infant. A heartbeat recording can be embedded onto a compact disc or thumb drive, or even put into a stuffed animal for a family to take with them and cherish. The heartbeat recording, whether with music or not, is a unique symbol of the patient. It is one of their defining characteristics, especially in infants.

Preliminary research suggests that heartbeat recordings do have an impact on the grieving process for bereaved caregivers.[15] Grieving and bereavement are both subjective and unique experiences for every individual, and bereaved individuals cope in varying ways; however, continuing bonds theory proposes that maintaining a connection with the deceased may be a helpful aid in coping. Heartbeat recordings are a continuing bond because they promote a sense of connection and bring back positive memories of their loved ones. Their use has been reported in this study as a means of connection, expression, and a helpful coping mechanism; however, with the heavy impact of its use, further investigation is needed to ensure the emotional safety and well-being of bereaved parents and caregivers.

CLINICS CARE POINTS

- The loss of an infant or child may be one of the greatest stressors a parent endures.
- Experts on grief and bereavement rely heavily on the continuing bonds theory to help understand the way bereaved individuals cope with the loss.
- Legacy-building and memory-making interventions have become increasingly popular in pediatric health-care settings, most recently in the NICU.
- Heartbeat recordings are being used as a legacy-building intervention and involve the use of a digital stethoscope to record an individual's heartbeat. In collaboration with a music therapist, live or prerecorded music may be added to the heartbeat recording.
- Heartbeat recordings can be considered a continuing bond in their ability to create and sustain a connection with the deceased.
- Health-care providers should consult a specially trained music therapist before introducing a heartbeat recording to a patient and family.

DISCLOSURE

The author has nothing to disclose.

REFERENCES

1. The National Center for Fatality Review and Prevention. Keeping kids alive: child death review in the United States, 2020 [Data Set]. Michigan Public Health Institute; 2021. https://ncfrp.org/wp-content/uploads/Status_CDR_in_US_2020.pdf.
2. Institute of Medicine (US) Committee on, In Field M.J. and Behrman R.E., Palliative and End-of-Life Care for Children and Their Families. When Children Die: Improving Palliative and End-of-Life Care for Children and Their Families, 2003, National Academies Press (US); Washington, DC.
3. Rogers CH, Floyd FJ, Seltzer MM, et al. Long-term effects of the death of a child on parents' adjustment in midlife. J Fam Psychol 2008;22(2):203–11.
4. Seigal C. Bereaved parents and their continuing bonds: love after death. Philadelphia, PA: JessicaPublishers, Kingsley Publishers; 2017.

5. Klass D, Steffen E. Continuing bonds in bereavement: new directions for research and practice. Routledge: Taylor & Francis Group; 2018.
6. Boles JC, Jones MT. Legacy perceptions and interventions for adults and children receiving palliative care: a systematic review. Palliat Med 2021;35(3):529–51.
7. Schaefer MR, Wagoner ST, Young ME, et al. Healing the hearts of bereaved parents: impact of legacy artwork on grief in pediatric oncology. J Pain Symptom Manag 2020;60(4):790–800.
8. Clements-Corte's A. Brian Schreck and the preliminary effects of music therapy cardiography. Can Music Educat 2017;58(2):34–6.
9. American Music Therapy Association. Music Therapy with Specific Populations: Fact Sheets, Resources & Bibliographies | Selected Bibliographies | American Music Therapy Association (AMTA). (n.d.). https://www.musictherapy.org/research/factsheets/.
10. American Music Therapy Association (AMTA). What is Music Therapy? 2023. Available at: https://www.musictherapy.org/about/musictherapy/. Accessed November 30, 2023.
11. Ghetti CM. Music therapy as procedural support for invasive medical procedures: Toward the development of music therapy theory. Nordic Journal of Music Therapy 2012;21(1):3–5.
12. Schreck B, Economos A. Perinatal music therapy: using Doppler recordings to connect and create. International Association for Music & Medicine 2018; 10(1):22–5.
13. Walden M, Charley.Elliott E, Ghrayeb A, et al. And the beat goes on: heartbeat recordings through music therapy for parents of children with progressive neurodegenerative illnesses. J Palliat Med 2021;24(7):1023–9.
14. Corrigan M, Keeler J, Miller H, et al. Music therapy and family- integrated care in the NICU: using heartbeat-music interventions to promote mother-infant bonding. Adv Neonatal Care 2021;22(5):E159–68.
15. Polara N, and Harman E. The Experience of Heartbeat Recordings for Bereaved Parents of Hospitalized Pediatric Patients. (Unpublished data, 2023).
16. Love A, Greer K, Woods C, et al. Bereaved parent perspectives and recommendations on best practices for legacy interventions. J Pain Symptom Manag 2022; 63(6):1022–33.

Maintaining Parental Roles During Neonatal End-of-Life Care: A Review of the Literature

William Cody Bartrug, MA, BSN, RN, RNC-NIC

KEYWORDS

- Neonatal intensive care unit • End-of-life care • Family-centered care
- Bereavement • Neonatal death • Meaning-making

KEY POINTS

- Bedside nurses facilitate building the parent-infant relationship by encouraging effective communication, building trust, and promoting parental role in end-of-life care.
- Effective communication is established by having open and honest dialog, providing clear and accurate information, and actively listening to the parents during end-of-life care.
- Building trust during end-of-life care requires consistency, support, empathy, compassion, and transparency with parents.
- Supporting the parent-infant relationship provides comfort and support to the dying neonate and long-term support and healing for the parents.

INTRODUCTION
Mortality

In the United States, the infant mortality rate is 543.6 for every 100,000 live births[1] with rates up to 40% in certain high-risk populations such as extremely low birth weight infants.[2] The neonatal intensive care unit (NICU) provides care to these high-risk populations and assists in the transition to end-of-life (EOL) care. With the rise in the importance of family-centered care within the NICU, parental involvement has become a crucial aspect of neonatal care. Neonatal nursing has adapted to this shift, but more improvement can be accomplished particularly with preparing for neonatal death.

Attachment Theory

Using attachment theory as a framework,[3] nurses can begin to understand the nuances of relationship building between parents and their baby. With advancing medical technology, parental relationships begin earlier during the prenatal period.[3] The

Intensive Care Nursery, UCSF Benioff Children's Hospital, University of California, 1975 4th Street, San Francisco, CA 94143, USA
E-mail address: william.bartrug@ucsf.edu

Crit Care Nurs Clin N Am 36 (2024) 289–294
https://doi.org/10.1016/j.cnc.2023.11.008
0899-5885/24/© 2023 Elsevier Inc. All rights reserved.
ccnursing.theclinics.com

relationship continues to build and grow until the expected delivery date. However, with a traumatic event such as a life-limiting diagnosis or an adverse event during delivery, the impact has great significance on the relationship due to the loss of the expected future.[3]

Parents often feel the loss of their parental role during an admission to the NICU[4] which can become exacerbated by the transition from curative care to EOL care.[5] The loss of this expected role can create a shift in the parents' meaning-making opportunities during the event of neonatal death.[6] "Meaning-making" allows parents to process the traumatic event and reorient their global meaning (ie, beliefs) which is central to their work of grieving.[7] Bereaved parents have higher levels of adverse health outcomes compared to the general population.[8] Therefore, it is imperative to understand the parental role during neonatal EOL care to provide appropriate support and enhance the overall care experience for these vulnerable families.

AIM

This review aims to explore relevant research around parental roles during EOL care in the NICU. This author identifies the role of the nurse in building and maintaining the parent-infant relationship.

DISCUSSION

The parental role in neonatal EOL care is of utmost importance due to the unique challenges and emotions that parents face when experiencing the loss of their child in the NICU.[9] Research has shown that involving parents in EOL care and decision-making processes can greatly improve support for parents and facilitate their ability to make informed decisions about the care of their infant.[10] This involvement should begin early on, during the prenatal period, and continue throughout the NICU stay. Parents should be seen as partners in care, with their input and preferences guiding the decision-making process.

Nurses play a key role in supporting parents during neonatal EOL care in the NICU.[11] They can use attachment theory as a framework to understand the dynamics of the parent-infant relationship and help foster a strong and supportive bond. Attachment theory during EOL care involves the recognition of the parent-infant relationship and the importance of maintaining and nurturing this bond, even in the face of a loss.[3] This can be done through effective communication, building trust, and promoting parental involvement in caregiving activities.[5]

Effective Communication

Effective communication can be achieved by fostering open and honest discussions with parents, providing them with clear and accurate information about their child's condition and prognosis, and actively listening to their concerns and preferences.[11] Open and honest discussions with parents involve acknowledging the emotional impact of the NICU environment and providing emotional support and encouragement to help parents overcome their fears and engage with their baby.[12] Clear and accurate information can be given to parents by providing updates on their infant's status, explaining medical procedures and treatment options, and discussing potential prognoses and outcomes. Being clear and accurate in communication helps parents understand and make sense of the situation, reducing uncertainty and anxiety.[5]

Active listening is an essential skill that allows nurses to truly understand the thoughts, emotions, and concerns of parents during this difficult time. By actively listening, nurses can validate parents' feelings and provide them with emotional support. Additionally, nurses should create an environment where parents feel comfortable expressing their emotions and asking questions. This can be done by creating a safe and non-judgmental space where parents are encouraged to share their thoughts and fears.

Building Trust

By engaging in open and empathetic communication, healthcare providers can establish a relationship of trust with parents, which is crucial for parental decision-making and overall support during neonatal EOL care. Building trust is accomplished by establishing a consistent and supportive relationship with parents, demonstrating empathy and compassion, and being transparent in all interactions. Furthermore, nurses can provide emotional support to parents, helping them navigate the complexities of the NICU environment, and cope with their fears and anxieties.[13] Additionally, nurses can play a crucial role in providing parents with EOL education and guidance.[11] This includes discussing treatment options, discussing the potential outcomes and prognosis, and providing resources and support for parents to help them make decisions that align with their values and beliefs.[14]

Promoting Parental Involvement

Promoting involvement in caregiving activities can also help parents feel a sense of purpose and connection with their child during EOL care.[5] This can include activities such as skin-to-skin contact, feeding and bathing their infant, reading or singing to them, and participating in care planning discussions. When parents are actively involved in these caregiving activities, they report feeling more connected to their child and more prepared for the EOL process.[5]

Nurses can further support parents in their role by providing education and guidance on the physical care needs of their infant, such as pain management, comfort measures, and symptom control. Pain management during EOL care can be particularly challenging in neonatal patients, as their ability to communicate discomfort is limited. Educating parents on cues and signs of pain in their infant, as well as providing them with information on various pain management strategies, can empower parents to play an active role in ensuring their infant's comfort and quality of life during this difficult time.[15]

In addition to providing emotional support and education, nurses can also advocate for parents' rights and preferences in the neonatal EOL care setting. This includes ensuring that parents are involved in decision-making processes, respecting their cultural and religious beliefs, and advocating for their wishes regarding the care and treatment of their infant. Nurses should also consider the unique needs and experiences of each family when providing EOL care. These may include factors such as previous experiences with loss, cultural and religious practices, and individual preferences for the timing and manner of EOL care.[5]

Meaning-Making

Meaning-making is the process by which individuals find or create meaning and purpose in their experiences.[6] During neonatal EOL care, parents often seek meaning in their child's life and death. They may engage in activities such as creating memory keepsakes, sharing their child's story with others, participating in rituals or ceremonies, or finding solace in spiritual or religious beliefs. Additionally, legacy building or memory-making by recording their child's heartbeat with or without music has been used in NICUs. Heartbeat recordings offer a material memento or treasure to parents. They can hold these recordings or other mementos close or share them with family and friends to sustain the continuing bond that has hopefully been created.[16] Healthcare providers, including nurses, can support parents in their search for meaning by actively listening to their thoughts and feelings, encouraging them to share their experiences, and providing a supportive and non-judgmental environment. A crucial part of this support is acknowledging their baby as a unique individual who had a meaningful existence, regardless of how short it may have been. This can include calling the baby by their given name and using inclusive language, such as referring to the parents as "mom and dad" or "parents."[17]

In the period after the death of their child, parents may experience intense grief and a range of complex emotions. These may include feelings of sadness, anger, guilt, and even relief.[18] By providing opportunities for relationship-building and promoting their roles as parents during EOL, they can utilize the process of meaning-making to navigate their grief and find a sense of purpose and value in their experiences. This can positively affect their mental health and well-being in the long term.[7] Thus, promoting the relationship between the parents and their infant not only provides comfort and support for the dying neonate, but long-term support and healing for the parents.

LIMITATIONS

The field of neonatology is vastly changing through research and innovation. However, research on EOL care and the support of families during EOL care in the NICU is very limited. Some limitations of this research article include the lack of comprehensive studies in neonatal nursing specifically focusing on parental roles during neonatal EOL care. This literature review was accomplished by integrating research from multiple disciplines.

Implications of Practice

The findings of this study have important implications for healthcare practices in the NICU. Firstly, it emphasizes the importance of involving parents in the care and decision-making process for their neonate(s). Parents should be given opportunities to actively participate in their baby's care, such as bathing, dressing, and changing them. This involvement not only affirms their role as parents but also allows them to create meaningful memories with their baby, even in the context of EOL.

Secondly, healthcare providers should prioritize effective communication and trust-building with parents. Open and honest communication between healthcare providers and parents is crucial to provide accurate information and address any concerns or questions that parents may have. This can help alleviate parental anxiety and provide them with a sense of empowerment and confidence in their decision-making.

Lastly, providing education to nurses on EOL care is vital in improving support for parents during this difficult time. Nurses should receive training on how to provide EOL care and how to support grieving parents, just as you would with any other competency. By equipping nurses with the knowledge and skills needed to navigate EOL care discussions and provide compassionate support, they can better meet the unique needs of parents during this sensitive and challenging period.

Implications of Research

Future research should continue to explore the parental role during neonatal EOL care, with a focus on understanding how healthcare providers can enhance and support parental involvement and decision-making during this sensitive time. By conducting more in-depth qualitative interviews with parents who have experienced neonatal loss, researchers can gain a deeper understanding of their experiences and perceptions regarding EOL care. Additionally, studies can investigate the effectiveness of specific interventions and programs aimed at supporting parents during neonatal EOL care, such as palliative care programs. Furthermore, research should also explore the impact of cultural and socio-economic factors on parental involvement in neonatal EOL care.

SUMMARY

The role of nurses in supporting parents during infant EOL care in the NICU is crucial. By developing partnerships with parents, nurses can provide the necessary support and guidance to navigate this difficult journey and build the relationship between parents and their child. Nurses can facilitate this relationship building by effectively communicating, building trust, and promoting the parental role. Effectively communicating requires open and honest dialog, clear and accurate information, and active listening. Building trust can be accomplished by providing consistency and support, empathy and compassion, and being transparent. Promoting the parental role allows parents to actively participate in EOL care through thoughtful education and guidance on the process of dying. As a result, parents will be able to rely on the experiences created and set up the process of meaning-making to grieve and cope with the loss of their infant.

CLINICS CARE POINTS

- Effective communication during end-of-life care is having an open and honest dialog, providing clear and accurate information, and actively listening.
- Building trust during end-of-life care is providing consistency and support, empathy and compassion, and being transparent.
- Promoting parental role during end-of-life care is educating and encouraging active participation in the dying process.
- Maintaining the parent-infant relationship supports and improves comfort for infants and improves long-term outcomes for parents.

DISCLOSURE

The author declares no conflicts of interest.

REFERENCES

1. Infant Health. (2023). National Center for Health Statistics; Center for Disease Control and Prevention. Available at: https://www.cdc.gov/nchs/fastats/infant-health.htm.
2. Patel RM, Rysavy MA, Bell EF, et al. Survival of infants born at periviable gestational ages. Clin Perinatol 2017;44(2):287–303.
3. Robinson M, Baker L, Nackerud L. The relationship of attachment theory and perinatal loss. Death Stud 1999;23(3):257–70.
4. Zaichkin J, editor. Newborn intensive care: what every parent needs to know. 3rd edition. American Academy of Pediatrics; 2009.
5. Baughcum AE, Fortney CA, Winning AM, et al. Perspectives from bereaved parents on improving end-of-life care in the NICU. Clinical Practice in Pediatric Psychology 2017;5(4):392–403.

6. Park CL. Meaning making following trauma. Front Psychol 2022;13:844891.
7. Neimeyer, editor. Meaning reconstruction and the experience of loss. Washington, DC: American Psychological Association; 2010. p. 261–92.
8. Harper M, O'Connor RC, O'Carroll RE. Increased mortality in parents bereaved in the first year of their child's life. BMJ Support Palliat Care 2011;1(3):306–9.
9. Bry A, Wigert H. Psychosocial support for parents of extremely preterm infants in neonatal intensive care: a qualitative interview study. BMC Psychol 2019;7:76.
10. Soltani Gerdfaramarzi M, Bazmi S. Neonatal end-of-life decisions and ethical perspectives. J Med Ethics Hist Med 2020;5(13):19.
11. Eden LM, Callister LC. Parent involvement in end-of-life care and decision making in the newborn intensive care unit: an integrative review. J Perinat Educ 2010. https://doi.org/10.1624/105812410x481546.
12. Thornton R, Nicholson P, Harms L. Being a parent: findings from a grounded theory of memory-making in neonatal end-of-life care. J Pediatr Nurs 2021;61:51–8.
13. Turner M, Chur-Hansen A, Winefield H. The neonatal nurses' view of their role in the emotional support of parents and its complexities. J Clin Nurs 2014; 23(21–22):3156–65.
14. Dagla M, Petousi V, Poulios A. Neonatal end-of-life decision making: the possible behavior of Greek physicians, midwives, and nurses in clinical scenarios. Int J Environ Res Publ Health 2021;18(8):3938.
15. Benoit B, Cassidy C, van Wijlen J, et al. Co-development of implementation interventions to support parent-led care for pain in infants: protocol for a qualitative descriptive study. JMIR Res Protoc 2022;11(8):e33770.
16. Polara N. The experience of heartbeat recordings for bereaved caregivers of hospitalized pediatric patients. Master's thesis. Philadelphia, PA: Temple University; 2023.
17. Lizotte M-H, Barrington KJ, Sultan S, et al. Techniques to communicate better with parents during end-of-life scenarios in neonatology. Pediatrics 2020; 145(2):e20191925.
18. Prins S, Linn AJ, van Kaam AHLC, et al. Diversity of parent emotions and physician responses during end-of-life conversations. Pediatrics 2023;152(3). e2022061050.

Printed and bound by CPI Group (UK) Ltd, Croydon, CR0 4YY

03/10/2024

01040471-0012